C000088131

PLANT-BASED DIET

HOW TO LOSE WEIGHT, IMPROVE YOUR
HEALTH AND MAKE PLANT-BASED DIET A
LIFESTYLE
30+ Delicious and Easy to Make Healthy Recipes

Stephan Nelson

PLANT-BASED DIET

REVERSE DISEASE, RESET YOUR BODY AND BURN FAT ENDLESSLY
30+ Delicious and Easy to Make Healthy Recipes

Stephan Nelson

CONTENTS

CHAPTER SEVEN: COOKBOOK

Image Credits: Shutterstock.com

INTRODUCTION

Now is the time to choose a diet that both nourishes you and limits the number of calories that you consume in a day. Is it possible to flood your body with nutrients and not calories? Yes, it is! One of the main contenders for nutrition and weight loss success is the plant-based diet.

What is a plant-based diet? Do you need to eat special foods? The plant-based diet is a diet that is rich in foods that come from plants. You do not need to buy special foods for this diet, but you might be new to some of the ingredients of a plant-based diet. For example, quinoa and millet are whole grains that you may not be familiar with yet.

What exactly do you eat on a plant-based diet? Some people think that a plant-based diet is vegetarian, but it doesn't have to be. First, it is important to decide what type of plant-based foods you are going to consume and if you are going to add any animal-derived foods such as meat, dairy, or fish to your diet. Whatever you decide to include in your diet, the main focus should be on eating foods that come from a plant source.

Let's look at the basic principles of a whole-foods, plant-based diet:

- Always eat foods that are whole and minimally processed.
- Avoid or limit animal products.
- Focus on eating fruits, vegetables, whole grains, seeds, nuts and legumes.
- Exclude refined sugars, white flour and processed oils.
- Include foods that are locally sourced and organic when possible.

(Kubala, 2018)

Not only will this book be about plant-based diets but I would like you to learn about whole foods. What is a whole food? A whole food is a food that remains close to its natural state when you eat it. (Dolson, 2020). For example, eating foods that do not have any added flavorings, added sugars, starches or manufactured ingredients. (Dolson, 2020)

Whole foods are important because they do not have a lot of additives that may cause you to become addicted to the food. Eating whole foods is also known as 'eating clean'. For a food to qualify as a whole food it needs to be as close to its natural state as possible. You will be learning a lot about whole foods in this book.

Can plant-based foods also be whole foods? Yes, they can. Most plant-based foods are consumed in their natural state. For example, plant-based foods such as fruits and nuts are usually eaten raw and unadulterated. Other plant-based foods like legumes, whole grains and beans are cooked but eaten without additives like sugar or other manufactured flavorings.

In this book, you will not only be learning about plant-based diet principles but you will also be going on a variation of the Body Reset Diet. The Body Reset Diet is a 15-day eating plan that concentrates on cutting down calories and consuming highly nutritious foods, and it is ideal for weight loss.

The Body Reset Diet was developed by a celebrity trainer, Harley Pasternak, who has a background in nutritional science and exercise physiology. He designed the Body Reset Diet as a vehicle for rapid weight loss. Pasternak believed that if he could jumpstart a person's weight loss, they would be more motivated to follow a weight-loss diet.

Pasternak also stuck to food plans that required very little time to be spent in the kitchen. In this book we will also provide easy no-hassle recipes to follow. The goal for the Body Reset Diet is for you to consume roughly 1,200 to 1,400 calories a day. This breaks down to 300 calories per smoothie, 150-200 calories per snack and 360 calories per meal. (Meixner, 2020) Pasternak also designed his diet to include non-taxing exercises to keep one motivated to exercise while following his weight loss diet.

Do you feel that you are not as healthy as you could be?

Perhaps you are eating foods that are detrimental to your health. I'd like to help you feel a lot healthier than you do now. This book will be your comprehensive guide to changing your diet. Not only will I recommend foods to add to your diet, but I will also recommend foods that you need to avoid such as salt, oil, and sugar.

Salt/Sodium

In many countries, salt is found on the dining table. The amount of salt you add to your foods is a personal preference, and many of us liberally indulge in adding salt to our meals. Yet, can going without salt actually be more healthy?

When you follow a whole food, plant-based diet, you will consume 400-600 milligrams (mg) of sodium daily from plant-based foods that naturally contain sodium. (Naked Food, 2020) The body does need sodium but there is really no reason to add extra table salt to your diet.

If you consume a low-sodium diet, you will realize many health benefits. For example, when on a low-sodium diet, your "intestines increase sodium absorption and the kidneys reduce the loss into the urine." (Naked Food, 2020) If you are on a high salt diet, this alters your sodium balance and your kidneys begin to reduce their functionality and remove less water. This adds to higher blood pressure and puts a strain on your kidneys and can lead to kidney disease. Not only does salt add to kidney strain but persons who consume a high amount of sodium often have kidney deterioration. (Naked food, 2020)

When people who have severely damaged hearts and kidneys lower their sodium intake, this stops some of the damage that is occurring in these organs. (Naked Foods, 2020)

Low-sodium diets enhance weight loss because salt often triggers overeating. Specifically, low sodium foods are less palatable. Consequently, when a person is starting on a low sodium diet, they eat less. Also, processed foods are restricted on a low-sodium diet and these are the foods that are calorically dense and typically high sodium.

The recipes in this book will focus on not adding salt to your food and eating foods that are low in sodium.

Oils

Studies have found that all types of oils are bad for your health. There is a commonly held belief that olive, coconut, grapeseed and flaxseed are considered 'healthy oils'. Although these oils are considered healthy, there is evidence that oils, such as olive oil, reduce the blood flow in arteries by 31%. (Naked Food, 2020) Moreover, olive oil causes significant damage to endothelial cells inside of the arteries. This type of damage causes inflammation which often leads to atherosclerosis or hardening of the arteries. (Naked Food, 2020)

Vegetable based oils are pressed from plants but all of the nutritional value is stripped away from them. These oils are considered only fat and they are very high in calories per gram. For example, 14 grams of fat are found in a tablespoon of oil.

The problem with processed vegetable oil is that it injures the endothelial cells found in blood vessels. These special cells make a protective molecule of gas and nitric oxide, that protects blood vessels and is responsible for the smooth flow of blood within our vessels. Nitric oxide dilates or makes our blood vessels wider for the passage of blood and also inhibits the inflammation of the blood vessels and the formation of plaques within those vessels. (Naked Foods, 2020)

Even fats that are considered monounsaturated fats, such as olive oil, cause damage to the endothelial cells that are in arteries. The damage is not as pronounced as in the consumption of foods that have trans fats or saturated fats but the damage still happens.

Oil in general has a negative impact on blood vessels. Further, the consumption of oil also has an impact on lung function and oxygen exchange, the suppression of the immune system and leads to an increased risk of cancer. (Naked Foods, 2020)

In this book, I will recommend foods that are oil-free.

Sugar

Some say life is sweet, but is our diet too sweet? In America the average person consumes 77 grams of sugar per day, or 60 pounds of sugar annually. (American Heart Association, 2020) Children can eat up to 81 grams a day, which is 65 pounds annually. Beverages seem to be the highest contributor to sugar in our diet. Here's where it is found: 25% soft drinks, 11% fruit drinks, 3% sports/energy drinks and 7% coffee and tea.

There have been many studies that point to disastrous health results when a person consumes sugar. There is growing scientific evidence that table sugar and high fructose corn syrup can trigger health disasters like liver toxicity and other chronic illnesses. (Naked Food, 2020) Of primary concern is the effect of these sugars on one's insulin sensitivity. When the body is flooded with glucose, it decreases insulin sensitivity, which causes cells to have difficulty in processing glucose. Furthermore, processed sugar causes an increase in fat in the liver and this increase leads to fatty liver disease. (Naked Food, 2020)

It is possible for food to be sweetened naturally. I will show you how to include foods in your diet that are naturally sweet like dates, figs, prunes, cranberries and apples. Processed sweeteners play havoc on your digestive system so they will not be included in any of our recipes.

Get Started

When you start a whole foods plant-based diet, you might find that you miss the salt, oil, and sugar. However, if you learn to prepare food in a different way, you will be able to add flavors that you have never experienced before. Your taste buds will open up to the freshness of the food that you are eating. However, the transition may be rough at first if you are used to eating processed food. Fast food is often very high in sodium and other additives. Eating food with no salt is going to take some getting used to if you were a fast food regular.

A whole food, plant-based diet comes with a lot of change, but rest assured that these changes are well worth it. Some of the benefits of following a whole food, plant-based diet are better heart health, prevention of type 2 diabetes, weight loss and a good dose of cancer prevention. I will discuss the benefits in more depth in Chapter 1.

If you follow a whole foods plant-based diet, you may find there are some minor drawbacks. Depending on your lifestyle, going plant-based could take a lot of effort on your part.

If you are used to eating out for your meals, it may be a big change for you to find restaurants that support your whole foods, plant-based diet. When you find these restaurants, there might not be a lot of options. The lack of options may drive you to start eating more meals at home. When this happens, will you be up to the shopping, meal planning and cooking required? In this book, I will share with you some great whole food and plant-based options. However, it may require a lifestyle change if you are used to fast food and eating in restaurants. The amount of change is up to you - embrace the changes and you will be rewarded with better health.

Overall, there is nothing unhealthy about a whole foods plant-based diet, but changing to this diet might take a little more effort than you are used to taking when you satisfy your hunger.

Use this book as a guide and reference for not only changing your lifestyle but for eating healthier meals and losing weight. The whole foods, plant-based diet is not about what you are taking out of your regular diet but more about the foods that you are going to add. Not only will I explain the important aspects of a whole foods, plant-based diet but I will also show you how to ease your way into this new lifestyle. Later in the book, I will provide you with many recipes to prepare. This will make it easier to adopt this new way of life while furthering your weight-loss plan.

CHAPTER ONE: WHY GO ON A PLANT-BASED DIET?

FOLLOWING A WHOLE FOOD, plant-based diet is the best weight loss diet on the planet because you get to eat more, not less! One of the principles behind eating whole food and plant-based diets is that these foods are nutritionally dense and not calorie dense.

When a food is calorie dense it has a lot of calories per pound. For example, a pound of oil has 4,000 calories per pound so it is very dense. Compare this to a pound of blueberries that have a lower calorie density of 261 calories per pound. Fruits, vegetables, starchy vegetables, legumes and whole grains are high in nutrient density. If you eat a diet high in caloric density, you will automatically not gain any nutrient density. For example, you will get a lot more nutrients in a piece of fruit or vegetable compared to what you would get in a tablespoon of oil.

The Food Advantage

Another advantage to eating unprocessed foods like whole grains is that you get fiber that makes you feel fuller. The same goes with fiber-rich fruit and vegetables. So, it is wise to fill your plate with non-starchy vegetables because they are full of fiber and water and average only 100 calories per pound. (Forks and Knives, 2020) You can also add whole grains and legumes to your plate to create a nutrient rich meal that will make you feel very full and content.

In the last part of this book, I will give your recipes that are low in calorie density and high in nutrient density. You will begin to add more foods to your diet than the amount of foods that you are taking away.

Think of it this way: if you are counting calories and caloric density, how much fried chicken can you eat? Not much - perhaps just a wing and a drumstick. Now think of how much whole food you can have on your plate that is low in caloric density and high in nutrient density. Think perhaps of a huge plate filled with your favorite fruits and vegetables and a bowl of savory quinoa. The sky's the limit when you choose nutrient density over caloric density.

All of this information may be hard to grasp at first but I will go into further detail and explain it fully. To make it easy, I will give you food plans that you can follow as you are getting to know more about the whole food, plant-based diet.

The Key to Losing Weight

A plant-based diet is ideal for losing and maintaining a healthy weight as it deals with foods that are not dense in empty calories. Eliminating processed and refined foods knocks out a lot of high caloric foods. Also, plant-based foods do not play havoc on your blood sugar. With the exception of some high-carbohydrate fruits, a plant-based diet can help with insulin sensitivity since many of the foods are high in fiber.

Once you become familiar with the foods that are included on the whole foods plant-based diet, you can begin to mix and match different tastes and textures that will fulfill your dietary needs. It will be hard at first to go without ingredients like salt, oil and sugar, but as time passes, you will begin to notice that your excess weight is dropping off. This is because you will no longer be eating foods that are calorically dense.

The key to losing weight is for you to eat whole foods that have not been tampered with. This will be a challenge in the beginning but imagine how many calories you're saving by eating whole foods that are unadulterated.

There are many diets that are popular right now. The problem with these diets is that they restrict the amount of foods that you can choose from. The key to being successful on any diet is to have many choices to choose from. We all have unique tastes and sometimes when we try to go on a diet, we have to force ourselves to eat the foods that are recommended on that diet.

The plant-based diet is a program that adds foods into your

diet. You will not be restricting anything other than animal-based products. Available to you will be the entire world of whole foods. Fruits and vegetables will become your favorites as you learn to prepare them in different and interesting ways.

Trying to eat foods in their purest form can be a challenge but it isn't anything impossible to do. It's just a new way of looking at food and food preparation. When you clear your palate of processed and sugary foods, you will be able to distinguish flavors that were absent to you before.

The effort that it will take to prepare whole foods will be well worth it. The health benefits that you will get from eating a healthful diet will make any extra effort you put forth well worth it.

The Flexitarian Diet

When one thinks of a whole food, plant-based diet, you usually think of a vegan or vegetarian diet. There is nothing wrong with that, but it is not always true. If you need a framework for your diet, you can follow a vegan or vege-tarian plan. However, you may feel that this type of diet is too restrictive for you. If this is the case, you may add non-plant-based diet foods like fish and poultry to your diet. The main thing is to flood your diet with plant-based foods. This is why the plant-free diet is often called the 'flexitarian diet' - because you can be flexible.

A plant-based diet isn't just about eating fruits and vegetables. Here is a list of foods that you can eat on a plant-based diet:

- Vegetables
- Fruits
- Whole grains
- Nuts
- Seeds
- Beans
- Lentils
- Coffee
- Tea

Foods to Avoid or Limit

Foods that you may want to avoid or limit are the following:

- All animal products
- eggs
- dairy (milk, cheese, etc.)
- red meat (beef, pork, etc.)
- poultry (chicken, duck, etc.)
- fish
- Processed animal meats (sausage, hot dogs)
- Refined grains
- Refined flours
- Refined sugars
- Sodas and other sweetened beverages
- Potatoes

- Honey

Some of these foods, such as sugar, may not be obvious animal-based products. Sugar is filtered with bone char, which is powdered animal bone. There may be an exception to this if you live in other countries besides the United States. For example, many leading brands of sugar in the UK do not contain bone char. (Nagesh, 2018) Check the labels carefully to find out if your sugar is vegan or not.

Overall, you get to choose what you want to include in your plant-based diet. Whether you go vegan or follow a diet that has some animal products, be sure to pick nutritionally dense foods.

VEGETARIAN DIETS VARY

There are many different types of vegetarian diet examples to follow:

- Lacto-vegetarians exclude meat, poultry, eggs, fish, and any foods that contain them. However, they do eat dairy products like milk, cheese, yogurt and butter.
- Ovo-vegetarians don't eat meat, poultry, seafood or dairy products, but they allow eggs.
- Lacto-ovo vegetarians exclude meat, fish, and poultry, but they allow dairy products and eggs.
- Pescatarians eat fish, but exclude meat, poultry, dairy and eggs.

- Vegans exclude meat, poultry, fish, eggs, dairy products, foods that contain these products and anything derived from animals.

(Mayo Clinic Staff, 2020)

The recipes in this book will closely follow the vegan diet.

The benefits of following a whole food, plant-based diet are many. In the next section we will examine what happens to the body when you stop eating meat.

BENEFITS TO ELIMINATING Meat from Your Diet

Lower Blood Cholesterol Levels

When you have an elevated blood cholesterol level, you are at a great risk for heart disease and stroke. A big culprit in elevating your cholesterol levels are saturated fats that are found in cheese, meat, poultry, and other animal products. (McMackin, 2016)

When you begin a plant-based diet, you eliminate these culprits and switch to eating legumes and complimentary whole grains in order to give your body protein.

Studies have shown that people who follow a plant-based diet experience a drop in their cholesterol levels of up to 35%. In some of these cases, these people are able to decrease the drug therapies that they use to prevent the buildup of cholesterol.

Two factors that help people lower their cholesterol levels when they follow a plant-based diet. There is less saturated fat and cholesterol in the foods that one eats on this diet. Furthermore, a plant-based diet is also high in fiber which reduces blood cholesterol. (McMackin, 2016)

THE REDUCTION of Inflammation in Your Body

When you eat a lot of meat, cheese and highly processed food, it is very likely that you have high levels of inflammation in your body. Inflammation usually happens when you have an injury, but this type of inflammation is short term. However, the inflammation caused by animal products is long term and has been linked to atherosclerosis (hardening of the arteries), heart attacks, strokes, diabetes and autoimmune diseases. (McMackin, 2016)

When you follow a plant-based diet, you do not experience a lot of long-term inflammation. In fact, plant-based diets have natural anti-inflammatory properties. The reason for these natural properties are because a plant-based diet is high in fiber, antioxidants and other phytonutrients.

HEALTHY MICROBIOMES

In our body there are a trillion microorganisms responsible for our gut health. These microorganisms are collectively called a microbiome. These microbes help to digest our food, produce critical nutrients, turn genes on or off, keep gut tissue healthy, protect us from cancer and train our immune systems. (McMackin, 2016)

When you are on a plant-based diet, you will have a healthy microbiome due to the fiber that is consumed in plant foods. People that eat animal products may have an unhealthy gut microbiome compared to people that eat a plant-based diet.

You can change your gut microbiome easily in a few days by getting on a plant-based diet.

THE GENE CHANGER

We depend on our genes to optimize cell repair damage and lengthen our telomeres (the caps at the end of the chromosomes that keep DNA stable). When you consume the antioxidants and other nutrients found in plant-based diets, you can enhance the repair of cell damage and telomeres. In fact, studies have shown that a plant-based diet decreases the expression of the cancer gene in men with low-risk prostate cancer. (MacCracken, 2016)

TYPE 2 DIABETES and the Plant-based Diet

The first thing that may come to your mind when you think of type 2 diabetes is carbohydrates because diabetics are advised to not eat a lot of carbs. However, eating meat is also harmful to those with type 2 diabetes. There are several reasons that meat is not good for a type 2 diabetic. Animal fat and animal-based iron and nitrate preservatives in meat cause damage to pancreatic cells, cause weight gain, impair the function of insulin and worsen inflammation. (McMackin, 2016)

So often we reach for something sweet without thinking of what these sugary snacks are doing to our body. There is a delicate balance between the insulin that is released into your bloodstream and the cells in your body. It's important that you do not impair this healthy balance by over-doing it with sugar and processed foods.

THE EFFECTS of Excess Proteins

There is a popular belief that protein makes a human stronger and leaner. This may be the case but when you have an excess of protein, it either turns to fat or into waste. This being the case, the excess protein is a cause of cancer, inflammation, diabetes, heart disease and weight gain. (McMackin, 2016)

When you are on a plant-based diet, you will have a healthy microbiome due to the fiber that you consumed from plant foods. People that eat animal products may have an unhealthy gut microbiome compared to people that eat a plant-based diet.

However, you need to stay away from processed vegan foods that imitate meat, such as vegan hamburger patties or hot dogs. Even though there is not any meat in these products, they are very processed and not good for you.

Remember, it is the quality of the foods you eat that will make the difference in your weight loss efforts.

When you eat a plant-based diet, you can decrease the damage caused by eating the wrong types of food. Foods like whole grains help protect against type 2 diabetes. (McMackin, 2016) In fact, the carbs that you eat in a plant-based diet can improve or even reverse your diabetic symptoms. (McMackin, 2016). In the case of a plant-based diet, carbs can be good for you if you get them from the right foods.

A POWERFUL EFFECT

Plant-based foods such as whole grains, beans, nuts, seeds, fruits and vegetables can have a powerful effect on the health of our bodies. In fact, there are many whole foods that can reverse unhealthy conditions in the body. Overall, when you go on a plant-based diet, you set up your body to heal and treat some of the damage that has been done by eating a diet full of processed food and animal products.

THE HEALTH BENEFITS of a Plant-based Diet

What are the advantages of a plant-based diet over a regular diet of restricting calories? A plant-based diet does not concentrate on the calorie content of the whole foods recommended for the diet. Instead, there is an effort to eat nutritious foods that help deter symptoms or illnesses that can happen when you don't pay attention to what you are eating.

If you are just counting calories and not paying attention to what you eat, will this help your body? No. For example, if you are only counting calories you could have a meal like fried fish and chips and max out your calories for the day.

Then you fast for the rest of the day so that you won't go over your calorie count. However, where is the nutrition?

If you are on a plant-based diet, you can pile your plate high with whole foods and know that you won't have to fast because the whole foods that you are eating are low in calories and will be digested in a healthful manner.

What's more, the plant-based diet helps to treat and prevent several major illnesses. Here are some examples:

Lower blood pressure - A meta-analysis study in the journal: *JAMA Internal Medicine*, April 2014, concluded that those who follow a plant-based diet have lower blood pressure on average compared to patients that included meat into their diet. Further, a November 2016 study published in the *Journal of Hypertension* found that patients who followed a plant-based diet had a 34% lower risk of developing high blood pressure compared to those who did not follow this diet. (Lawler, 2020)

Heart health - A study published in the *Journal of the American Heart Association*, August 2019, came to the conclusion that a plant-based diet reduces the risk of developing cardiovascular disease by 16%. In particular, eating whole grains, vegetables, fruit and legumes add to your heart health as these healthy foods substitute for foods that are incredibly harmful. (Lawler, 2020)

Prevention of type 2 diabetes - It is well known that type 2 diabetes is linked to a person's food choices or diet. A 2016 study reported in the *PLOPS Medicine* journal found that the risk of developing type 2 diabetes goes down 34% when you follow a plant-based diet. A study published in *Diabetes Care* reported that the prevalence of type 2 diabetes was only 2.9% for vegans and 7.6% for non-vegans. (Lawler, 2020)

These are just a few of the benefits that come from following a whole foods, plant-based diet. Weight loss is also a big benefit to following a whole foods, plant-based diet.

There are many benefits to following a diet that is crammed packed with foods that are not processed and meat based. One of the major benefits is weight loss. The whole-foods, plant-based diet is more like a way of life than it is a restrictive diet. Choosing to eat foods that are not processed rules out eating fast-food but not eating out. You just have to choose your meals wisely. Instead of eating a traditional hamburger, try a vegan burger instead. If they are 'homemade' or made 'in house' the patty will be made from whole grains and legumes. Avoid the pre-made processed vegan meat substitutes you can buy at the store, as they are packed with ingredients you don't need.

PLANT-BASED Diets and Chronic Diseases

There is evidence that a plant-based diet can prevent and cure chronic diseases like cardiovascular disease, obesity, and certain cancers. According to an Institute of Food Technologist (IFT) study, people who live in a society that follows a plant-based diet rarely experience chronic diseases. Discoveries in nutritional genomics explain why plant-based diets ward off diseases. (IFT, 2020)

The World Health Organization (WHO) reports that 63% of deaths in 2006 were caused by chronic diseases such as cardiovascular disease, certain cancers, obesity, and type 2 diabetes. (IFT, 2020)

An example of the positive results of following a plant-based diet are that the antioxidants in plant foods counter free radicals that are responsible for chronic inflammation and cell damage. Furthermore, "plant compounds help control a gene that is linked to cardiovascular disease and plaque buildup in arteries and the genes and other cellular components responsible for forming and sustaining tumors." (IFT, 2020)

Foods like artichokes, black pepper, cinnamon, garlic, lentils, olives, pumpkin, rosemary, thyme and watercress, just to name a few plant-based foods, may play a major role in preventing cancer and other chronic diseases.

Weight Loss and The Plant-based Diet

When you eat whole foods, you add a lot of fiber to your diet and this helps you feel full and consequently, you tend not to overeat when you are eating whole foods. The key seems to be the fiber in a plant-based diet. Fiber takes longer to digest so you feel full longer. Consequently, you begin losing weight because you are not over-eating.

A review of literature in the *Journal of General Internal Medicine* found 12 studies done with 1,150 people who went on various weight loss plans for 18 weeks. The people on a plant-based diet lost an average of four pounds more than those people who ate meat on their diets. (Fowler, 2020)

The study also found that people on a plant-based diet stayed on the diet longer than their counterparts that ate meat in their diets. (Fowler, 2020)

ENERGY BOOST on a Plant-based Diet

There are many reasons why a plant-based diet boosts your energy levels. One obvious reason is that your digestive system is working at peak efficiency. Also, you are meeting your body's macronutrient needs. As soon as you switch to a plant-based diet, your body begins to repair itself, so there will be a point where you have prevented and cured certain chronic illnesses.

The true boost to your energy levels when on a plant-based diet are the vitamins like vitamin B6. Foods that contain vitamin B6 are bananas, sweet potatoes, squash, walnuts, spinach, kale, avocados and peanut butter. What does vitamin B6 do? Vitamin B6 helps you to rest and relax as it regulates nervous system activity. When you meet your B6 needs you will probably get a good night's rest. Consequently, you will wake up in the morning very rested and full of energy. (One Green Planet, 2020)

If that isn't enough, remember that your body is maintaining a healthy sugar level so there will be no spikes in blood sugar that will make you 'crash'. This combined with the fact that it takes less energy to digest the foods on a plant-based diet ensures that you will increase the energy available to do many things. In essence, you will have a constant boost of energy.

Following a plant-based diet can reverse disease, reset your body and help you achieve weight loss easily. It is amazing the impact that eating a healthy, whole food, plant-based diet can have on your health.

Chapter Summary

- Following a whole food, plant-based diet is the best weight loss diet on the planet because you get to eat more, not less.
- One of the principles behind whole food, plant-based diets is that these foods are nutritionally dense and not calorie dense.
- If you are not ready to go vegan and want to keep some animal products in your diet, be sure to pick nutritionally dense foods.
- When you begin a plant-based diet, you eliminate the bad sources of animal protein and switch to eating legumes and complimentary whole grains in order to give your body good protein.
- You can change your gut microbiome easily in a few days by getting on a plant-based diet.

In the next chapter you will learn more about how to incorporate the plant-based diet into your life.

CHAPTER TWO: A PLANT-BASED DIET FOR BEGINNERS

TRANSITIONING from a regular diet to a whole food, plant-based diet will be the best thing you will ever do for yourself. It might be tough to leave behind some of the foods that you are accustomed to. Who doesn't love a hamburger or a hot dog? What about pizza? Will you have to say goodbye to the pizza pie?

It may be hard at first but you can make your transition to a whole food, plant-based diet easy if you take it in stages. You may be saying goodbye to Chicken McNuggets and fast food as you know it, but you are gaining a lot of great foods. Think of your transition as gaining a whole lot of health instead of thinking about the meat, dairy and eggs that you are giving up.

Every transition has steps. There is no reason to go quick and rough when it comes to making the transition. Take it slow and be patient with yourself. Here are some steps that will make your transition easier.

START With Just One Day

Before transitioning completely to a whole food, plant-based diet, try to schedule one day a week to follow the whole food, plant-based diet. Many people start with meatless Mondays. Your body needs to get used to the increase in fiber and plant-based proteins. Starting with just one day also helps you to start small with the new way of cooking. For example, you can learn to cook cauliflower in a way that will be delicious and different. Craving wings? Try some buffalo cauliflower with blue cheese dressing. You might find that you aren't missing a thing.

The good thing about cooking a plant-based diet is that plants can last longer than some meats so you will have more flexibility about what you are cooking. Beans, a whole grain, last longer than chicken breasts or ground meat that needs to be frozen to increase its shelf life.

Another part of the transition is more fiber. When you begin to take in the fiber of beans, whole grains, fruits and vegetables, your body needs to adjust. Doing this one day a week is a very good way to start. You can start with just one day and then keep adding days until your whole week is meatless.

SWITCH-OUT DAIRY for Non-dairy Products

Dairy has been a part of your life since you were a baby and now you are making a decision to no longer have dairy in your diet. This might be a very tough choice for you depending on how much dairy you already consume. However, the transition may not be as hard as you think. There are many plant-based dairy alternatives such as non-dairy yogurt, nut milk-based beverages and vegan cheese.

You may find the transition easy because these plant-based substitutes are very much like their dairy counterparts. For example, almond, cashew or soy milk is very much like cow's milk. In fact, these milks often come in sweetened vanilla flavor to make the transition easier. Non-dairy yogurt is also a favorite. You can also add fruit to your non-dairy yogurt to make it more appealing. Vegan cheeses are much like their counterparts as they come in blocks and sliced forms. There are hard cheeses and soft cheeses. You can even find nacho cheese to put on your chips.

CHEESE ALTERNATIVES ARE MADE From Different Sources

Food source alternatives for cheese are soy, tree nuts and seeds, coconut, flour, root vegetables and aquafaba. You can find many different flavors of cheese to suit your palate. All in all, the switch from dairy to non-dairy can be very satisfying.

LEARN to Cook Your Favorites With Plant-based Alternatives

It can be hard to say goodbye to some of your old favorites like chicken wings, macaroni and cheese and pizza but did you know that with a little creativity, you can make your favorites out of plant-based alternatives?

All you need to do is learn to be more creative in choosing your ingredients. Foods like cauliflower can be cooked in different ways such as seasoning it to make cauli-wings or using nutritional yeast to make the cheese in your mac-and cheese dish. By blending cashews, carrots, potatoes and nutritional yeast, you can make a pretty tasty and presentable mac and cheese dish.

A bonus with plant-based foods is that with the added fiber, you will feel full quicker and stay full longer. Plus, you might feel delightfully lighter as you are not bogged down with heavy non-plant-based foods.

Make Plant Protein the Star of Every Meal

If you've spent a lifetime eating meat and animal products, it might be hard for you to switch to plant-based proteins. The good news is that plant-based protein like beans and whole grains can be very filling. Think vegan chili or white bean pizza.

Are you worried that you won't be able to get enough protein in your diet? If you make plant-based protein the star of every meal, you shouldn't have a problem. There are many dishes that we will introduce in this book that will meet and exceed your protein requirements. The good news is that plant-based food has a lot of fiber and this will make you feel satisfied and full a whole lot longer than your traditional protein meals.

PLANT-BASED PROTEINS

Until you started reading about plant-based protein, you might have never thought such a thing existed. After all, we are brought up eating meat, poultry and fish. However, there are many different types of plant-based protein. Here is a list of some plant foods that contain protein.

Beans like chickpeas, kidney, black and pinto beans are very high in protein. Beans and chickpeas contain 15 grams of protein per cooked cup. Also beans and legumes decrease cholesterol, lower blood pressure, reduce belly fat and help control blood sugar levels. (Petre, 2016)

Green peas are a surprising source of protein. They have 9 grams of protein per cooked cup. The little green pea also serves up 25% of the daily requirement for fiber, vitamin A, C, K, thiamine, folate and manganese. (Petre, 2016)

Lentils are a super source of protein as they contain 18 grams of protein per cooked cup. Lentils are also a really great source of fiber. A single cup of lentils contains 50% of your recommended fiber intake. Lentils are rich in folate, iron, manganese, and are an antioxidant. (Petre, 2016)

Nutritional yeast is a deactivated strain of Saccharomyces

cerevisiae yeast that is sold as a yellow powder or flakes. Nutritional yeast has a cheesy flavor and is a popular ingredient in plant-based foods as you can sprinkle it on pasta or enjoy it on popcorn. Nutritional yeast is an excellent source of protein as it provides 15 grams of protein per ounce.

Seitan is made from gluten that is the main protein in wheat. (Petre, 2016) When you cook seitan it has the texture of meat. Seitan contains 25 grams of protein in a 3.5 ounce serving. It is also a good source of selenium, iron, calcium, and phosphorus. When shopping for food, you will find seitan in the refrigerated section of your store. You can pan-fry, sauté and even grill seitan.

Tofu, tempeh, and edamame are whole protein sources from soybeans and as such provide your body with all the essential amino acids. (Petre, 2016) Tofu really doesn't taste like anything so it is a good candidate for mixing with other foods to absorb their tastes. Tofu is bean curds pressed together similar to the way that they make cheese. Tempeh originates from tofu but it is cooked and fermented from mature soybeans and is pressed into a patty. Tempeh has a nutty flavor. Edamame is great to snack on. It's an immature soybean with a sweet and grassy taste. You can steam or boil edamame and eat it alone or add it to your soups and salads. Tofu, tempeh, and edamame all contain iron, calcium and 10-19 grams of protein per 3.5 ounces. (Petre, 2016)

ADD, Don't Subtract When Planning Your Plant-Based Meals

Frame of mind is very important when you are making the transition to following a plant-based diet. You might be overwhelmed with all the foods that you can't eat, but a plant-based diet is more about the foods that you are going to add to your diet.

Think about getting 5 to 7 servings of fruits and vegetables a day – then add the protein you will be eating with every meal – that's a lot more food than you are probably used to. Yet, this is what you are going to be eating from now on.

There are many new foods for you to try such as tofu, tempeh, seitan, and a broad variety of legumes. Mealtime will now be an adventure as you transition to a plant-based diet. Your plate is going to be piled high with delicious foods.

Fill Up Your Plate

When you begin to transition, start with filling up half your plate with vegetables. You may still be eating chicken and beef but you can start trying the variety of vegetables that you will be adding to your diet. For example, along with your eggs, you might add avocados and tomatoes to your plate.

Not only are vegetables and fruits an excellent source of vitamins, minerals and antioxidants, they are also beautiful on your plate. Think of the bright color of tomatoes and carrots – the resplendent colors of salad greens like kale and spinach. Who wouldn't like such a vibrant plate of food?

A very popular plant-based food item these days are the food bowls that mix together whole grains, fruits and vegetables and legumes. You can also grill your fruits and vegetables as a new taste for your palate. If you start adding plant-based foods to your plate as you are transitioning, the faster you will be acquainted with your new diet.

The Right Way to Cook Plant Protein

Tofu and tempeh will become the cornerstone of your plant-based protein choices. If you don't learn to cook tofu and tempeh properly, you might be eating undercooked and under-seasoned food that will really turn you off. Learning to season and cook these plant-based proteins isn't hard. With just a little bit of effort you can have some pretty awesome tasting plant-based protein meals.

Tofu is tasteless until you season it. Tofu can take on any flavor that it is exposed to. Consequently, it is a very popular plant-protein to use. Don't be discouraged about cooking plant-proteins. There are many plant-based proteins recipes that we will share in this book that are crazy-delicious.

Don't Be Afraid to Ask

When you are making the transition to a plant-based diet, you might find it challenging to eat out. There are more and more restaurants that are offering plant-based diet meals. However, there are still some restaurants that have not caught on to this trend. What can you do? Well, don't be afraid to ask if you can have a substitution to your meals. For example, the restaurant may add foods to your plate like tofu or beans. You can also get some pretty amazing salads if you just ask. Remember it is not about what you subtract from the meal but about what you can add. Partner with your waiter to build a tasty plant-based meal. All you have to do is ask.

BUILD Healthy Meals

It can be a new experience to build meals for yourself. If you have spent years on bacon and eggs for breakfast, it will be a big change for you to eat something plant-based like non-dairy yogurt or tofu cooked like eggs. You might even get frustrated when trying to think of meals that you can prepare.

Breakfast and lunch menus can be a challenge when you are on the go. Save the difficult recipes for supper-time and for fixing meals in the evenings for use the next day. Get very creative with building your meals. Instead of a sandwich at lunch, try a plant-based salad with a whole wheat like quinoa. There are many foods that you can prepare on-the-go. You might have to learn to prepare your foods ahead of time, but it will be worth it.

FRESH OR FROZEN?

When you think of a plant-based diet, fresh fruit and veggies come to mind, but have you ever thought of buying frozen fruits and vegetables? From a whole foods perspective, it is best to eat fresh but sometimes that won't be possible. Make it easy on yourself and have frozen fruits and vegetables for those times that you are in a hurry.

It isn't always possible to have time to scrape carrots or chop broccoli. If you have a stash of frozen vegetables in your freezer, you're one step closer to having food on the table. Make your transition easier by choosing recipes where you can use frozen fruits or vegetables.

Think "flash-frozen" when you shop for frozen fruits and vegetables. These types of frozen foods can be just as nutritious as fresh and sometimes even more so when you think of produce that has been brought to your store from a farm that is far away.

Frozen produce can also be easier on your pocketbook, and that is important when you are making your transition. Plus, if you are starting with only one day or two a week, frozen produce will keep longer than fresh.

Frozen fruits are very important if you like to make a lot of smoothies. When fruit prices are fluctuating, or fresh fruit is unavailable, a stash of frozen fruit will serve many purposes.

It is good to go frozen for your smoothie ingredients. You can sometimes buy a large bag of frozen fruit for the same price as a quart of fruit like blueberries or strawberries. Plus, when you buy frozen, you don't have to worry about finding fruit when it is out of season or buy fruit that is going to spoil on you before you use it all up.

It takes no time to mix up a smoothie, and if the fruit is frozen you can get a very appealing texture in your smoothie. You can also add a protein powder or a nut butter to your smoothie so that you have that added protein.

Overall, buying frozen is not only good for your pocketbook but it makes your transition easier.

Play With Your Food

Making the transition into eating plant-based food is an invitation to play with your food. Foods that you never thought would go together, or foods cooked in a different way, can really change your perspective. If you are used to having boiled vegetables as a side-dish, rethink your side-dish to be steamed or sautéed vegetables instead. It's not only vegetables that can be cooked differently but you can take a food like yogurt and use it in a different way. For example, Indian dishes use yogurt as a sauce that quiets the heavy spices in the meal. Yogurt isn't just for breakfast.

Carve out vegetables like sweet potatoes or melons to hold a specially prepared dish. Mix two foods together that you have never had. For example, sweet potatoes and chickpeas mashed together and put in a sweet potato "boat" is really tasty.

Don't be afraid to play with your food and produce combinations that you have never tried before.

Have you ever thought of cooking with fruit juice instead of broth? Can you steam vegetables instead of boiling them? What about using spices instead of salt to cook a dish? Learning to cook whole wheat in delicious ways can add excitement to your dining experience too.

Learning to play with your food and finding different ways to prepare plant-based foods can really help your transition. Every transition has steps. Take it slow and steady, and be patient with yourself.

When you start eating a plant-based diet you won't always be at home. What happens when you are away from home? Is it possible to stick to a plant-based diet?

Eating Out

Here are some tips and pointers for sticking to your plant-based diet when you are eating out.

Be creative about what you order at a restaurant. Study the menu for plant-based options and order one if they have it. This will encourage the restaurant to keep items like that on the menu. If they don't have dishes that are specifically plant based, be creative. For example, a restaurant's main entree option usually comes with steamed vegetables. Order the steamed vegetables without the entre. Don't be timid about picking apart meals so that you end up with only plant-based food. Get creative and create one meal out of many meals. This can easily be done ordering from the appetizer, side-dish and salad menus. Also, you can ask if the cook would mind cooking you a plant-based meal.

Pick a restaurant that will have a lot of plant-based options. There are many vegetarian restaurants in major cities. Asian restaurants cook a lot of vegetables and may even have tofu on the menu. Before you head out to a restaurant, try to get a look at their menu online so that you know if they serve any plant-based menu items. If their menu is not on the internet, call ahead and ask if they prepare anything plant-based. Also ask if they would mind cooking something special for you.

Here are some suggestions of plant based foods that you will be able to order at a restaurant:

- Italian foods will have pasta and tomato sauce and steamed vegetables. Be sure to stay away from the cheese.
- Steakhouses usually have the best baked potato or sweet potato on their menu. They will also have steamed vegetables and large salads.
- Breakfast restaurants will probably have oatmeal available. Call ahead to see if they have any plant-based milk. You might also be able to order fresh fruits, whole grain bread and perhaps some kind of nut butter if available.
- Coffee shops usually have herbal teas along with their coffee. Many of these shops are now also serving plant-based milks and non-dairy creamers. Oatmeal is also a popular choice at coffee shops. Mix dried or fresh fruit into your oatmeal.
- Gas stations or convenience stores may carry foods like unsalted nuts or whole grain pretzels. These stores may also carry foods that are vegan.

- Grocery stores will have tons of plant-based foods. If you are traveling and pass a grocery store, be sure to stop. You can assemble a good picnic lunch and find somewhere nice to park and eat.
- Some grocery stores may have food bars where you can sit and eat. These often include a salad bar.

If you plan ahead and get creative you can follow your plant-based diet anywhere you go.

(Esselstyn, 2016)

OTHER FOOD OPTIONS

Packing your meals to-go is also an option. There are an assortment of lunch boxes and bags available that will accommodate your plant-based meals. Lunch boxes are no longer just for children! There is a strong market for adult lunch boxes that are insulated and easy to use. Rubbermaid has a Lunchbox salad kit that enables you to keep your salad fresh until it is time to eat. Look for lunch boxes that will suit your needs. If you want to just pack ingredients and fix your meal when you get to your destination, choose an insulated tote bag. Keep utensils and other miscellaneous items like napkins stored in your car or maybe in a reusable tote.

Foods like canned beans or dried fruit keep very well in your car. Buy a cheap can-opener to keep in the car for when you need a quick plant-based meal.

Following a Plant-based Diet

Two of the questions you need to ask when you are switching to a plant-based diet are: How strict are you going to be when following it? What is your motivation to follow a plant-based diet?

As you learned earlier, there are many different types of vegetarians and many reasons for choosing vegetarianism. Not all vegetarians are strict about not eating animal products. They are semi-vegetarian, or a variation of vegetarians that eat eggs, dairy and fish. There are people who follow a vegetarian diet because they want to improve their health. Others follow a strict vegan diet because they are concerned about the environment or the treatment of animals, as opposed to being concerned about their health.

In the last chapter you learned about the different types of vegetarians. In this chapter, let's take a look at the seven different types of diets more closely.

There are three types of vegetarians that include eggs and dairy in their diet. These types are:

- Lacto-ovo-vegetarian
- Lacto-vegetarian
- Ovo-vegetarian

The differences are as follows: Lacto-ovo vegetarians eat both eggs and dairy; lacto-vegetarians include only dairy; and ovo-vegetarians include eggs.

31

The next three types of semi-vegetarians include protein that is not plant-based:

- The pescetarian diet includes fish, eggs and dairy products.
- The flexitarian occasionally eats meat, fish and poultry.
- The pollotarian eats chicken and other poultry but no other types of animal products.

This leaves the vegan diet, which is the most pure form of vegetarianism. Vegans do not eat any type of meat product or any products derived from animals. This includes dairy, eggs or even honey. Vegans sometimes also choose not to wear animal products like leather.

Which type of vegetarian are you going to become? Why are you motivated to not eat animal products? Which animal products are you going to abstain from? These are all questions that should be answered so that you can fine tune your diet.

THE FLEXITARIAN DIET

The flexitarian diet is one of the easiest diets because you are flexible with what you can eat. If you want to incorporate meat, eggs or dairy in your diet for a meal or two, that's all right. If you do this, what about the health benefits of not eating animal products? Will you still receive the benefits if you are not strict about following a whole food, plant-based diet? When you eat meat products, eggs and dairy, there are consequences to your body, such as inflammation and increased cholesterol. It isn't so much that the whole foods, plant-based diet benefits are erased if you eat some animal products, it's just that you may not be eating enough of these foods to make a difference in your health. Are you willing to do without some of the benefits like losing weight, lower blood sugar levels, improved kidney function, protection against certain cancers and a lower risk of heart disease?

The Motivation to Change

Improved health is a strong motivator to become a vegetarian. Whatever type of vegetarian you choose to become, you might want to know the benefits to the environment and to the animals that you are saving because you are restricting your food to a whole food, plant-based diet.

Being sensitive to animal life is one of the major reasons that vegans refrain from eating meat. They feel that animals have emotions and an intelligence that ought to stop us from slaughtering them. Vegans feel that it is inhuman to slaughter an animal for food because animals are sentient beings. You will often hear a vegan say that they will not eat anything with a face.

Factory farming destroys many of our resources. More and more acres of natural land are being claimed by farmers. Deforestation and the drive to get more farmland is tearing apart the countryside.

Not only are farmers taking land to raise animals but they are also using up a huge amount of water for the animals they are raising for slaughter. Also, farmers are using pesticides on the crops that they are growing to feed their animals. These pesticides in turn get into the animals and we eat those animals and hence absorb the pesticides.

If we only ate a plant-based diet, the amount of land and resources to grow this type of food would be only a fraction of what farmers use now.

When you become a vegan who doesn't eat any animal products, not only are you saving factory animals but you are also saving the natural predators of the animals that are farmed. Coyotes, wolves and other predators are captured and killed by farmers to protect their stock animals.

If there was not a need to stock animals, the grain that these animals are fed could go towards feeding all those who are suffering from hunger in developing countries. The water being used for animals could be distributed to the agricultural areas where water is scarce.

Not eating meat products can also become a moral stance that extends to shutting down animal agriculture and channeling resources to other areas.

TRANSITIONING TO A WHOLE FOODS, Plant-Based Diet

Eating a whole foods, plant-based diet takes time for you to get used to. No matter what your passion is, you are going to need time to learn how to prepare plant-based meals and you are going to have to train your palate to new flavors.

It is not the end of the world if you become a flexitarian to begin with. Being flexible with what you are eating is a good way to start the journey into vegetarianism.

It might even be a good idea to try each of the seven different kinds of vegetarianism. You might systematically go through these types, giving up meat products a little at a time.

For example, you might just give up beef first and still eat fish and chicken. Then after you get used to that, you could give up chicken and just eat fish. At the same time that you are systematically giving up meat products, you can increase the quantity of whole foods and plant rich foods. You can begin to train your palate to new flavors. When your palate has changed, this may be the time to give up fish and only rely on dairy and eggs. Then after a while, eliminate dairy and include just eggs, and then after that only eat whole foods and plant-based foods.

ETHNIC FOODS

There are many ethnic foods like Indian or Asian foods that use spices in a different way than western foods. You can experiment with these foods and get used to not just tasting them but also preparing them. Also, there are many vegetarian dishes in other cultures, and we can learn a lot of great cooking ideas from exploring ethnic food.

IT'S GOING to be a big change for you at the market as you spend more time in the produce aisle buying up all the different vegetables and fruits that you will now be eating. It may take you 4-6 weeks or even a year to fully transition if you take your time to make the change. During this time you will begin to feel better physically as your body becomes more healthy. You might even experience more energy.

Becoming a vegetarian is a journey not a race. There may be a day that you really miss a good steak. So, go out for steak or cook at home. Just don't give up on vegetables and fruits. Maybe just have a few ounces of steak instead of a large whole steak. Pile your plate high with tasty vegetables. The same would go if you wanted to eat chicken or fish. Cut down your portion of the animal-based protein in order to increase the plant-rich foods that you can eat.

You will also find that you do not need as much salt, sugar or oil in your diet. Eliminating these three things can yield some amazing health results.

Whatever type of vegetarianism that you choose to follow, remember to be patient with yourself as you make the transition.

As you decide on eating a whole foods, plant-based diet, I would like to present to you a seven-day meal plan that will help you kick-off your diet. The following meal plan is inspired by and adapted from the 7-day plans on the website eatingwell.com.

Meal Plan - 7 days

Day 1

Breakfast

3/4 cup of oatmeal

1/2 cup strawberries

Snack

1 orange

Lunch

Carrot soup with crackers

Dinner

Veggie-topped pizza

Snack

Banana

Day 2

Breakfast

Tofu scramble with tomatoes and green chilies

Snack

Apple

Lunch

Whole-wheat veggie wrap

Dinner

Black bean burger and side salad

Snack

Hummus and fresh vegetables

DAY 3

Breakfast

Dairy-free yogurt with bananas and granola

Snack

Peach

Lunch

Tomato sandwich with pesto and drizzle of extra-virgin olive oil

Dinner

Spaghetti squash

Snack

Roasted chickpeas

DAY 4

Breakfast

Oatmeal with almond milk and chopped apples

Snack

Hummus with carrots

Lunch

Avocado toast

Dinner

Sweet potato stew

Snack

2 clementines

DAY 5

Breakfast

1 serving toast with mascarpone and berries

Snack

Bananas and cashew butter

Lunch

French onion soup

Dinner

Vegetarian chili with avocado

Snack

Handful of almonds

Day 6

Breakfast

Avocado toast

Snack

Apple and peanut butter

Lunch

Whole-wheat pasta and roasted tomatoes

Dinner

Quinoa bowl with roasted carrots and sweet potatoes

Snack

Non-dairy yogurt and strawberries

Day 7

Breakfast

Oatmeal with almond milk

Snack

Bananas with raisins and cashew butter

Lunch

Greek salad with slice of whole-grain pita bread

Dinner

Veggie burrito

Snack

Roasted chickpeas

CHAPTER SUMMARY

- Before transitioning completely to a whole food, plant-based diet, try to schedule one day a week to follow the whole food, plant-based diet. Many people start with meatless Mondays.
- Frame of mind is very important when you are making the transition into following a plant-based diet. You might be overwhelmed with all the foods that you can't eat but a plant-based diet is more about the foods that you are going to add to your diet.
- Making the transition into eating plant-based food is an invitation to play with your food. Foods that you never thought would go together or foods cooked in a different way can really change your perspective.
- Being sensitive to animal life is one of the major reasons that vegans refrain from eating meat. They feel that animals have emotions and an intelligence that ought to stop us from slaughtering them.

- When you become a vegan, not only are you saving animals, but you are making resources available for other types of food production.

IN THE NEXT chapter you will learn tips for starting your plant-based diet.

CHAPTER THREE: TIPS FOR BEGINNERS TO GET STARTED

Now THAT YOU are thinking seriously about going on a whole foods, plant-based diet, here are some tips that will help you to make your transition successful.

Eat lots of vegetables! This may seem like a 'no-brainer' but you are going to have to eat vegetables in place of other foods, like in the morning instead of eggs or at dinner time instead of steak. There are many vegetables that are versatile enough to be filling and satisfying. Cauliflower is a vegetable that can be substituted for rice or chicken.

Thinking about vegetables in a different way is going to help you make the transition more easily. This is where getting to know the food of other cultures will come in handy. Asians have some great recipes that use vegetables as the center of their meals. When it comes to Indian food, a good vegetable curry is very satisfying as an entree.

Fruit can be more than a dessert. You can add most fruits

into a salad to punch up the flavor. You don't just have to use lettuce and tomato for your salad. Pomegranate seeds and strawberries are sweet and tart enough for a salad. You can try any combination of fruit with your salad.

Desserts made primarily from fruit are also very satisfying. You can freeze bananas to make banana ice cream, or you can freeze peaches and melons to make an afternoon snack.

There is no limit to what you can do with fruits and vegetables.

KING of the Meal

For many years, meats have been the king of the meal. We have learned to grill it, pan fry it, and roast it to perfection. You might find that most of your recipes are about cooking meat, chicken and fish. How do you switch to plant-based protein when all you know how to cook is meat?

There are foods like tofu and tempeh that can be substituted for meat. These two plant-based proteins absorb the taste of whatever you are cooking it with. You can add sauces or spices to make these proteins taste good. You can make everything from tofu scrambled eggs to sweet and sour tofu 'chicken'.

Lentils are another food that has a lot of protein. Cooked lentils contain 8.84 grams of protein per 1/2 cup. Red or green lentils have an abundance of iron and potassium. You can add lentils to stews, curries, rice or even salads.

Chickpeas are another popular protein. They contain around 7.25 grams of protein per 1/2 cup. Chickpeas are the basis of hummus dips. You can add them to stews, curries or roast them in the oven and season with paprika for a crunchy snack.

Nuts like almonds and peanuts can add protein to your meals. Eat a handful of these nuts when you are too busy to fix a meal. A handful of these nuts have between 16.5 grams to 20.5 grams of protein per handful.

Other foods that are a good source of protein are:

- Spirulina (blue or green algae)
- Quinoa
- Mycoprotein
- Chia seeds
- Hemp seeds
- Beans with rice
- Potatoes
- Vegetables like leafy greens, broccoli and mushrooms
- Seitan
- Ezekiel bread

Eating Foods With Less Oil

After a lifetime of fried foods, it is time to start eating foods with less oil. It would be good to get rid of oil or fats in your foods all together but this can be tough. Start a transition to doing without oil by only using healthy oils. These oils and fats come from olive oil, olives, nuts and nut butters, seeds and avocados.

Get creative in the way you prepare your foods. If you want to follow a recipe for stir-fried vegetables for example, use olive oil. Just be careful of high heat because olive oil breaks down over high heat.

MEATLESS MONDAYS

Have you ever heard of meatless Mondays? This is where you serve a vegetarian meal for dinner every Monday. If you really want to challenge yourself, you can go the entire day only eating plant-based foods. Some families use meatless Monday to become more aware of vegetarian foods. Others use meatless Mondays to transition to eating a complete whole foods, plant-based diet. It's hard sometimes with a family to get everyone on the same page when it comes to changing your diet. Whoever is doing the cooking usually controls what is going to be eaten. There have been many family fights over a major change in diet. To not have this happen in your household, meatless Mondays is a good way to segue way into a plant-based diet.

There are many fantastic recipes, like cauliflower mac n' cheese, that are a good substitute for the foods you and your family love. Enjoy being meatless by building your meals around beans, whole grains and vegetables. Don't forget the fruit dessert!

This book includes some really tasty recipes you will learn to cook and enjoy.

TRADITIONAL FOODS

For years breakfast was dominated by eggs, bacon and toast. Walk into any diner and you will find every kind of egg combination imaginable. How do you go from something as traditional as scrambled eggs to a plant-based breakfast?

The way to do it is to become familiar with whole grains. Whole grains can be your friend at breakfast. There are many different ways to have these grains. Oatmeal is a traditional breakfast food and you can sweeten it by adding sweet fruits like apples or berries. Quinoa, buckwheat or barley are also whole grains that you can use to make something traditional like muffins. Many of these whole grains can be ground down to a flour.

Another ideal breakfast is one that is rounded out with the addition of seeds, nuts and fresh fruit. Sunflower seeds blend very well into your foods.

Whole grains are more filling because they are high in fiber. Think of a muffin made with whole grains compared to one that is made with only white flour. Not only will you feel more full but you won't experience a rise in your blood sugar. Whole grains take longer to be digested and made into glucose. A muffin with white flour and refined sugar is going to play havoc with your system. You might get a short burst of energy, but as your blood sugar climbs, you will start feeling a bit sick.

Stick to whole grains at breakfast for an energy that will last longer and feel good.

The Nutrients in Green Foods

Growing up, you may have told your mother that you didn't want to eat any food that was green. Your mother probably made you eat green food anyway because she knew there was a world of nutrition in green food. Leafy green vegetables like kale, collards, Swiss chard and spinach bring a lot of nutrition to the table. You can steam, grill, braise or stir-fry to keep the nutrition in the greens. Avoid boiling vegetables, as this leeches all the nutrients out of them.

Leafy greens bring many nutrients to the table, including vitamins C, A and K. They also are full of antioxidants, calcium, folate, iron and potassium.

Another big benefit from leafy greens is the fiber. Having fiber is very good for your digestive system. Leafy greens can be eaten raw in a simple salad. Mix greens together or concentrate on just one. Kale can also be roasted in the oven to make kale chips that can be seasoned with a little bit of salt.

If you do not like your greens raw, stir-fry is a good answer for preparing greens.

VEGETABLES FOR DINNER

Starting with vegetables for dinner can be easy or complicated. If you are pressed for time, think about building your meal around a salad. Serving foods that are in their most natural form is so very good for nutrition. You can do so many things with a salad. You can add fruit or whole grains to boost the nutritional value of the salad. You can add nuts and seeds to add a crunch and more protein to your diet.

There is a whole group of salads that were made around the humble bean. The three-bean salad is just one of them.

Salads are an excuse to use all the fruits and vegetables that you have in your kitchen. You can whip up a zesty or sweet salad dressing using fresh herbs and spices. You can marinate the tofu so that it has a specific flavor to enhance your salad.

A salad can feature a style or ethnicity of food. Mexican taco salad or Chinese chicken salad (without the meat of course) are good examples.

Buy a set of large salad bowls so that you can serve up those leafy greens, vegetables, fruits, nuts and seeds. Don't be shy about the ingredients you are using. Fill up a large serving bowl and let the salad shine.

THE FRESH FRUIT Dessert

Fresh fruit makes a great dessert when you are short on time. Shop for a large variety of fruit so that you can make amazing fruit salads. Spend time going through the produce section of your grocery store and get to know the fruit that your stores sell. If you don't have a wide variety of fruits in your local grocery store, go to an ethnic market to find fruits that you normally don't see in mainstream super markets. If you find a favorite, ask your grocer if they would consider stocking the produce department with some different fruits.

For lunches you can bust out of the same old fruit habits and pack melons or berries instead of an apple or orange. Cut the melons the night before so that they are easy to pack in the morning. You don't have to stick to just one kind of berry, try two or three types of berries for your non-dairy yogurt.

It's not a bad thing to go 'old school' and have a banana, apple or orange for desert. There are many different varieties of apples that you can try. There is the pink pearl, ambrosia, Arkansas black and good old winesap just to name a few varieties of apples. Citrus fruits also have some stars like blood orange, meyer lemons and clementines.

Become a fruit explorer and shake up your dessert time with exotic fresh fruits or stick to old school favs if you really like them.

Your Favorite Meals Turn Plant-based

A good place to start when you are transitioning into a whole foods, plant-based diet is to make a list of your favorite meals. Get in touch with the foods that are your favorites. Think of the tastes and textures of these foods. Then do some research on how to prepare some of these favorites as a meatless version. Think of vegetables like cauliflower and spaghetti squash that can be made into pretty good substitutes. Also very popular right now are the special cutters that can spiral cut vegetables like zucchini into noodles. These noodles can be eaten with a good sauce and you won't even miss the pasta.

You can also make new favorites. Tofu and tempeh are such great sources of tasty protein-packed meals. You can make these protein powerhouses into so many traditional or exotic dishes. It just takes a good imagination.

Sometimes your favorite foods can 'go vegan' and be purchased pre-made. However, be careful of buying vegan foods that are highly processed. You might be able to get hamburgers and hot dogs made from plant-based materials, but the nutritional value isn't as good, and it is far from being a whole food.

The key to changing into a whole foods, plant-diet is to add nutrition to your diet. Don't overthink your choices. Getting through the transition won't be as hard as you imagine. Make a trip to the grocery store or go to your grocer's website and investigate. Look for the foods that you see in plant-based recipes. Does your grocery store carry enough plant-based foods to keep you satisfied? You might need to supplement your shopping by going to a near-by farmer's market or an ethnic store.

The most important tip to follow when you are starting a plant-based diet is for you to eat as many whole foods as possible. The next tip is to develop a solid list of favorite foods as you encounter them.

Many people feel that following a plant-based diet is more of a lifestyle change than it is a diet. You are free to develop your own guidelines for the foods that you are going to eat. As discussed in this book, there are many different types of vegetarians. Perhaps you won't eat meat but perhaps you find it too hard to get rid of eggs in your diet. Or, you might want to stick with eating fish and other foods from the sea. Whatever you choose, just be sure to exclude foods with added sugars and refined oils. Keep in mind that a plant-based diet does not have to be as rigorous as a vegan diet.

The quality of the foods that you are eating are also very important. Choose foods that are locally sourced and organic at every chance. When you are making such a big effort to eat whole foods, make sure that you get food that is healthy and not weighed down with additional pesticides or other things that shouldn't be in your food.

Another tip to consider is if you are going to be adding any artificial sweeteners to your diet. There is a lot of controversy over the health and safety of these additives. It's up to you whether you include this sweetener into your diet. As you go through a detox plan, it is a good idea to avoid these sweeteners. Try other natural sweeteners before you make your decision. In fact, after you go through the detox diet, your palate might not need the added sweetener in your diet.

As you begin to try more and more foods, you might find it easier to stock your pantry with whole foods so that you are ready to cook up what you fancy on a whim. Here is a sample plant-based shopping list (Kubala, 2018):

- Beverages: coffee, tea, sparkling water, etc.
- Condiments: vinegar, lemon juice, salsa, mustard, nutritional yeast, soy sauce, etc.
- Fruits: bananas, peaches, berries, citrus fruits, plums, etc.
- Healthy fats: avocados, olive oils, unsweetened coconut oil, etc.
- Legumes: peas, chickpeas, lentils, black beans, etc.
- Plant-based protein: tofu, tempeh, seeds, nuts and nut butters including almonds, cashews, macadamia nuts, etc.
- Spices, herbs and seasonings: basil, rosemary, turmeric, curry, sea salt, etc.
- Starchy vegetables: potatoes, sweet potatoes, squash, etc.
- Unsweetened plant-based milks: almond, coconut, cashew, soy
- Vegetables: spinach, cauliflower, carrots, kale, broccoli, peppers, etc.
- Whole grains: quinoa, whole wheat pastas, brown rice, rolled oats, etc.

AFTER YOU SHOP

The best thing you can do for yourself is to prepare foods for your diet as soon as you get home from the grocery store. Specifically, wash and cut up vegetables and store them in the order that you will be using them for the week.

It's also a plus if you can store the items that you will need for a recipe together in the same place in your cupboard or pantry. You can pre-measure the spices that you will be using and put them in small containers or small reusable bags.

The more you do in preparation for cooking, the easier you will have it when it is time to prepare the meal. If there are foods that you can cook ahead, do this so that when you get really hungry, you have something that you can instantly prepare or heat up.

DEVELOP **Your Own Tips**

Take a look at the 14-day Detox Plan and the recipes ahead of time. This way you can already be thinking of the things you can do to make this plan go easier for you. There may be new ways to prepare food or even foods that you have never prepared before. A little bit of research can go a long way.

Remember, the easier you make things happen, the more likely you will stick with a plant-based diet that is new to you.

CHAPTER SUMMARY

- Stick to whole grains at breakfast for an energy that will last longer and feel good.
- Leafy greens bring many nutrients to the table such as vitamins C, A and K. They also are full of antioxidants, calcium, folate, iron, and potassium.

- The key to changing to a whole foods, plant-diet is to add nutrition to your diet, and minimize meat and other animal-based products.

IN THE NEXT chapter you will learn about the foods that you need to avoid and the foods that you can eat on a plant-based diet.

CHAPTER FOUR: WHAT TO EAT, LIMIT AND AVOID

WHEN YOU FEEL you are ready to start a whole food, plant-based diet, it is important to know the foods that you can have and the foods that you can't have. The best way to think about this type of diet is to focus on the foods that you can have. You will find that the list of the foods you can have is a lot longer than the foods that you can't have. In this chapter let's take a closer look at the diet and why it is one of the most nutritious diets to follow.

Whether you choose to follow a vegan-type diet where you don't have any meat products or you decide to be a flexitarian, the most important thing is that each food that you do eat is packed with a lot of nutrition.

PLANT-BASED PROTEIN

First let's start with plant-based protein. One of the go-to categories for protein are legumes. They are a healthy option that are full of iron and protein. Lentils and beans, for example, contain 10-20 grams of protein per cooked cup.

Legumes are also a great source of antioxidants, fiber, iron, folate, manganese and zinc. To absorb more iron and zinc from legumes, it is important to sprout, ferment and cook the legumes in a way that will help increase the absorption of nutrients.

Lentils are a legume that contains 18 grams of protein and fulfills 50% of your daily fiber intake needs. Lentils feed the good bacteria in your colon. They also contain folate, manganese, antioxidants and iron.

Chickpeas are very high in protein and fiber. They average about 15 grams of fiber per cup. They are an excellent source of iron, folate, phosphorus, potassium, manganese.

Overall, beans and legumes lower your cholesterol, blood pressure and blood sugar levels. You can even reduce your belly fat by eating beans and legumes.

SEEDS AND NUTS for Protein

Another great source of protein is seeds, nuts and nut butters. A 1 ounce serving of seeds or nuts contain as much as 5-12 grams of protein. Seeds and nuts are also an excellent source of fiber, iron, magnesium, zinc, vitamin E and selenium.

THERE ARE some seeds that have a greater amount of protein than others. Chia seeds, flax and hemp seeds are very high in protein. 1 ounce of hemp seeds for example, contains 9 grams of complete protein. Seeds are also rich in alpha linolenic acid.

It is best to buy nuts and seeds that are raw and unblanched. Blanching can affect nutrients in nuts and seeds. It's also wise to buy nut butters that do not contain oil, sugar and a high amount of salt.

OTHER SOURCES of Plant-Based Protein

Seeds, nuts and legumes are not the only good sources of plant-based proteins. Available to you are minimally processed meat alternatives like tofu, seitan or tempeh. These can sort of be thought of as mock meats because you can cook them in a way to taste like meat substitutes. In particular, Asian foods with their unique sauces can be cooked with tofu, tempeh, or seitan.

Seitan is a product that is made from the protein in wheat called gluten. It can be pan-fried, sautéed and grilled. Seitan contains 25 grams of protein per 3.5 ounces. It is also a good source of selenium. Seitan is one of the most rich plant-based sources of protein.

Tofu and tempeh are made from soybeans and provide the body with essential amino acids because it is a complete protein. Tofu and tempeh have 10-19 grams of protein per 3.5 ounces. Tofu is made by pressing bean curds together and tempeh is made from soybeans that are cooked and slightly fermented. Tempeh usually is made into a pressed patty.

Related to tofu and tempeh is edamame, which is an immature soybean that is steamed, boiled, or eaten on its own. You usually find edamame in soups or salads or as a salted snack.

A seed that has a lot of nutrition are chia seeds. They have 6 grams of protein per 1.25 ounces and are a good source for iron, calcium, selenium, magnesium, omega-3 fatty acids and antioxidants.

You may find that these little seeds are bland when you taste them. They become a gel-like substance like tapioca when they absorb water. You can put chia seeds in smoothies and baked goods. A popular way to eat chia seeds is to make puddings out of them.

Dairy and the Plant-Based Diet

When you go on a whole food, plant-based diet, you not only have to pay attention to your protein consumption but also the amount of calcium in your diet. Giving up dairy can be something that is difficult for you but there are substitutions that taste just as good as dairy.

Plant-based milks like almond, soy or cashew can be a very tasty alternative to cow's milk. Non-dairy yogurts are also a good alternative to dairy as they are a good source of vitamin D and B12.

Soy milk is a great substitute for cow's milk. Soy milk has 7 grams of protein per cup and is a great source of calcium, vitamin D and vitamin B12. Some soy milks are not fortified with B12 so pay attention to the nutritional values printed on the carton.

Other Foods High in Nutrients

A food that you may have never thought of eating is seaweed. Why should you consider eating seaweed? Well, it's a very good source of protein, fatty acids, antioxidants, and iodine. Another food that you don't think of eating is nutritional yeast, but it is a protein-rich source of B12.

Spirulina is also another food that you don't ever think of eating. Spirulina is a blue-green alga that is a nutritional powerhouse. Two teaspoons of spirulina has 8 grams of complete protein and 22% of the requirements of thiamin and iron. It also has 42% of your daily copper requirements. You can also find a healthy dose of magnesium, manganese, potassium, and essential fatty acids in Spirulina.

Spirulina is also good for you because it has anti-cancer fighting properties and anti-inflammatory properties. It is also known to reduce blood pressure, help regulate blood sugar and boost your immune system.

Wild rice is another food that is off the beaten path. It is an excellent source of protein, containing 7 grams in a cooked cup. Wild rice is a good source of fiber, manganese, magnesium, copper, phosphorus and B vitamins.

Be cautious and pay attention to the source of the wild rice as arsenic sometimes accumulates in the bran of the rice due to its being cultivated in polluted areas. Make sure and wash the wild rice and use a lot of water when you boil it, to get rid of some of the arsenic if you are worried about it.

NUTRITIOUS FOODS Already in Your Pantry

Some high-protein foods that are not very exotic but are found in our cupboards are green peas and oats.

Green peas are very versatile but mostly find their way into our diet as a side-dish. Green peas are a super source of protein because they have 9 grams of protein per cooked cup. The pea has 25% of the daily requirement of manganese, folate, thiamine, fiber and vitamins A, C and K. You can also find zinc, copper, phosphorus, magnesium and iron in green peas.

Another common pantry food is oats. They are a good source of protein, coming in at 12 grams of protein and 4 grams of fiber per cooked cup. Oats are also known to be a complete protein and a good source of magnesium, zinc, phosphorus, and folate. Oats are often eaten as a breakfast food but it also can be ground into flour and added to baked goods.

FOODS that Surprisingly Contain Protein

Fruits and vegetables can also contain protein. Vegetables that contain 4-5 grams of protein per cup are broccoli, spinach, asparagus, artichokes, potatoes, sweet potatoes and brussel sprouts. Fruit containing 2-4 grams of protein per cup are guava, mulberries, blackberries, nectarines and bananas.

Surprisingly, sweet corn, which is often classified as a grain, contains 4-5 grams of protein per cup.

Proteins that come from a plant-source come with a lot of added nutrients that our body needs. The best thing about these plant-based proteins is that they have a powerhouse of nutrients per cup. It is clear that farming these plant-based proteins is not as hard on the earth as raising animal proteins.

WHOLE GRAINS and Complex Carbohydrates

Another important food category to add to your whole foods, plant-based diet are whole grains that are complex carbohydrates. Grains such as teff, and the ancient grain spelt contain more protein than rice and wheat. Also, pseudo cereals like quinoa and amaranth are super grains that contain almost 9 grams of protein per cooked cup.

Ancient grains are ancient forms of what we think of as our modern grains. These ancient grains are sometimes thought of as a 'superfood' because they are packed with more nutrients than their modern-day counterparts. Ancient grains also have a good hearty taste.

Mostly grown organically, ancient grains can replace any modern grain in a recipe. Spelt for example, is an ancient grain that is ground into a flour that is a lot like our common modern-day wheat flour.

Ancient grains have not been altered like our modern-day grains. Modern day grains have been modified over the centuries by farming techniques and science. Ancient grains have retained valuable nutrients because they haven't been stripped down during the agricultural process.

Ancient grains are higher in protein, omega-3 fatty acids, antioxidants, vitamins and minerals compared to modern grains. There are even some ancient grains that are gluten-free. Even the grains that are not gluten-free seem to be more digestible than their modern counterparts.

There are 12 ancient grains that are used commonly today. They are: amaranth, barley, buckwheat, bulger, faro, freekeh, kamut, millet, quinoa, sorghum, spelt and teff.

THE BENEFITS of Whole Grains

The benefits of including whole grains in your diet are many. The most important fact is that whole wheat has a lot of fiber and this fiber helps you to feel full when you are eating. Whole wheat can also help you to keep your blood glucose levels down. Don't confuse whole wheat with its stripped down 'relatives' like regular flour.

Whole wheat is a whole food because it is delivered in its most original form. You can do a lot for your diet if you just switch out refined foods like white bread and pasta with their whole wheat counterparts. Foods like whole grain pasta and rice are a lot better for you. Don't forget about the classic oatmeal or whole wheat bread. If you would like to really crank up your diet, the ancient grains and seeds can really boost nutrition.

Another whole food option that should be included in your whole food, plant-based diet are sprouted grains that are soaked and grown in environments with controlled amounts of moisture and warm temperatures. These whole-grain seeds sprouts can be processed at home or in a manufacturing plant.

Whether you go for ancient grains or just regular whole wheat foods, you will be improving your diet and feel full for a lot longer than if you eat foods that are refined. Bread, rice and pasta can be more nutritious if you eat the whole wheat version.

Ancient grains spelt, telf, barely, sorghum and farrow are very good sources of protein. Spelt and teff have 10-11 grams per cooked cup. These two are the highest in protein of the ancient grains. Spelt and telf are a complex carbohydrate that contain a lot of fiber, iron, magnesium, phosphorus, manganese, B vitamins and selenium. You can add these grains to foods like risotto, polenta and baked goods.

Amaranth and quinoa are pseudo cereals that contain 8.09 grams of protein per cup. They are known to be a complete source of protein on their own. They are also a source of complex carbohydrates, fiber, iron, manganese, phosphorus and magnesium. You can also grind these two ancient grains into flour or just use them the way you would use a traditional grain.

ADDING **Fruits and Vegetables to Your Diet**

Following a whole food, plant-rich diet has the benefit of being highly nutritious. After you learn to eat plant-rich protein, the next thing you need to do is add more fruits and vegetables to your diet.

Fruits and vegetables have a lot of nutrients that are so very good for your body. Let's look at some of the amazing health benefits of fruits and vegetables, starting with vegetables.

The nutrients in vegetables help keep a person healthy. Here is a list of vegetables and how they help us stay healthy:

- Antioxidant and anti-inflammatory benefits: asparagus
- Digestive health: asparagus, onions and garlic, red cabbage and squash
- Disease prevention: asparagus
- Eye health: beets, bell pepper, squash, sweet potatoes and tomatoes
- Heart health: beets, carrots, collard greens, turnip greens, kale and spinach, red cabbage, squash, sweet potatoes and tomatoes
- Cancer prevention: beets, broccoli, cauliflower, collard greens, turnip greens, kale and spinach, onions and garlic, red cabbage, squash and tomatoes

Fruits also contain some amazing nutrients that contribute to our well-being. Here is a list of some fruits and the good that they do for our bodies.

- Apples are great to eat as they help reduce asthma risk, regulate your blood sugar and lower your cancer risk.
- Apricots are good for eye health and heart health.
- Bananas help with heart health and help you maintain your blood pressure in a healthy zone. You can look forward to increasing your bone strength and also get some ulcer relief if you have ulcers.
- Blueberries are a super fruit as it gives you antioxidant support, brainpower boost, cancer protection, cardiovascular defense and helps you to maintain your blood sugar levels. Lastly, blueberries are good for your eyes and help you keep them healthy.
- Cantaloupe helps to energize you along with helping to boost your immune system. Cantaloupes are also good for your eye and lung health.
- Cranberries are up there with blueberries when it comes to keeping you healthy. Here are some things cranberries can do for you: anti-aging benefits, anti-inflammatory effects, increased heart health and keeping your urinary tract healthy.
- Grapefruits are good for cancer prevention, immune system support, kidney stone prevention and cholesterol support.
- Grapes really give a lot of benefits like anti-aging and anti-inflammatory benefits, blood sugar

regulation, cancer prevention and cardiovascular and cognitive health support.

- Kiwi fruit gives you asthma and DNA protection plus they are good for heart health. Unique to this fruit is the ability to help reduce macular degeneration risk.
- Lemons and limes are good for cancer prevention and rheumatoid arthritis prevention.
- Oranges support digestive health, respiratory health, and immune system health. Oranges also lower bad cholesterol and heart health improvement.
- Papayas are fantastic at providing cancer prevention, heart health, inflammation reduction and immune system health.
- Pears are good for our eye health and they are also very hypoallergenic and can be eaten safely by persons who are allergic to most foods.
- Pineapples help give you more energy and they support digestive comfort, and anti-inflammation. This fruit also gives you immune support.
- Plums are great when you need help with iron absorption and immune strength. Also look for cancer prevention from this fruit.
- Strawberries also help with cancer prevention and cardiovascular help. This fruit also helps to regulate your blood sugar and provides anti-aging benefits.
- Watermelons also have anti-aging benefits, prevent cancer, support eye health and give you an increase in energy.

Foods to Avoid

Even though there is a lot to add to your diet when you start a whole food, plant-based diet, there are also many foods to avoid. The obvious foods to avoid are meats, poultry, seafood, eggs and dairy. Here is a list to use when you as you are getting used to the idea of avoiding foods that are not plant-based:

- Dairy (including milk and cheese)
- Meat and poultry (like chicken, beef and pork)
- Processed animal meats, such as sausages and hot dogs
- Eggs
- Refined grains such as 'white' foods like white pasta, rice, and bread
- Sweets like cookies, brownies and cake
- Sweetened beverages such as soda and fruit juice

There are also foods that are not so obvious that you should avoid. Here are a list of some of those foods:

- Honey or any bee products
- Deep-fried foods that use eggs in the batter to coat the food
- Beer and wine beverages that use egg white albumen, gelatin or casein during the beer or winemaking process
- Olive tapenade that also uses anchovies
- Bean products that use lard or ham

- Non-dairy creamers that have casein, a protein that comes from milk
- Pesto that contains parmesan cheese
- Dark chocolate that uses animal products such as whey, milk fat, milk solids, clarified butter or non-fat milk powder (There are some dark chocolates that don't use these products so check the label.)
- Produce that has been coated with beeswax or shellac
- Bakery products like bagels and breads that contain L-cysteine, an amino acid from poultry feathers
- Caesar dressing that contains anchovies
- Candies like marshmallows, gummy bears, chewing gums and Jell-O that contain gelatin plus candies that are coated in shellac that contains carmine (a red dye made from cochineal insects)
- French fries or deep-fried food that is fried in animal fat
- Pasta made with eggs
- Worcestershire sauce that contains anchovies
- Roasted peanuts that have gelatin added so that spices and salt will stick better
- Refined sugar that is made with bone char that is a natural carbon and made from bones of cattle
- Potato chips flavored with powdered cheese or a flavoring that may contain casein, whey, or other animal-derived enzymes.

Vegan Foods to **Avoid**

There are even vegan foods that should be avoided when you are on a whole food, plant-based diet mostly because these foods are far from being in their natural state and therefore not whole foods. These foods are the following:

- Vegan sweeteners like molasses, date syrup and agave. These sweeteners should be used in small amounts. Added sugar in your diet is linked to heart disease and obesity.
- Mock meats and cheeses are processed foods that have a lot of additives.
- Vegan junk food like ice cream, candies, cookies and chips
- Dairy-free milks that contain sugar
- Vegan protein bars that have added sugar, especially refined sugar

Chapter Summary

- Overall, beans and legumes lower your cholesterol, blood pressure and blood sugar levels. You can even reduce your belly fat by eating beans and legumes.
- Another great source of protein are seeds, nuts and nut butters.
- Tofu and tempeh are made from soybeans and provide the body with essential amino acids because

it is a complete protein. Tofu and tempeh have 10-19 grams of protein per 3.5 ounces.

- Another important food category to add to your whole foods, plant-based diet are whole grains that are complex carbohydrates.
- Ancient grains are ancient forms of what we think of as our modern grains. These ancient grains are sometimes thought of as a 'superfood' because they are packed with more nutrients than their modern-day counterparts.
- Fruits and vegetables have a lot of nutrients that are so very good for your body.

IN THE NEXT chapter you will learn about the plant-based Reset Diet.

CHAPTER FIVE: PLANT-BASED RESET DIET

Now that you know what a plant-based diet requires, it is time to put your knowledge to action. The very first thing that you need to do is make a commitment to change the way you eat. In particular, you must commit to eating a plant-based diet. When you start a plant-based diet, your body is going to go through some changes. In this chapter and the next, we will focus on your reset.

What is a reset? Well, the first part of a reset is taking out the foods that are not good for you and replacing them with healthy versions such as zucchini noodles instead of regular pasta noodles or home-made vegan burgers versus beef hamburgers.

You might think that going on a plant-based diet is going to be all about the things you take out of your diet, but as mentioned before, the plant-based diet is about what you add to your diet. Add more leafy greens, more vegetables, more legumes and whole wheat.

You will also need to eat more frequently. That's right - you will have to eat MORE. When you reset your diet, you will be eating 5 times a day: breakfast, snack, lunch, dinner, dessert. This is because the foods you eat are not as dense and calorie intensive as when you were on a diet that includes animal products.

The reset diet plan is going to help add foods that are healing and help with the detox that occurs when you go without the food that was causing you damage. In fact, your metabolism will change due to the fact that you are eating a plant-based diet and not a high calorie-dense diet.

FOLLOWING the Reset Diet

While on the Reset Diet, you will begin to feel clear headed and very hydrated. You will also stop craving sweets. This is a major change for you because you will no longer be eating foods that require sugar to make the food sweet.

Think of the Reset Diet as spring cleaning. Even pro-vegans need a Reset Diet for a few days to get back to feeling good. Even vegans can fall prey to processed foods and foods that are calorie dense. So, don't be discouraged when you look at the plan for the first time and realize just how much you are going to have to change the way you eat.

Let's take a look at what you are going to be taking out of your diet: preservatives, colorings, salt, fat, flavorings and sugar. You will also be removing refined foods from your diet like white rice, white bread and regular pasta.

Focusing on Whole Foods

You will begin to focus on whole foods. Whole foods are food as close to its original form as possible. Think of how foods are processed and stripped down to an almost non-nutritive state. Rice comes with bran but when you eat white rice, the bran is stripped away. Think about the way we cook foods - when we peel, wash, dice, slice and fry foods. A potato is chocked full of nutrients but when it becomes fried, those nutrients are muted.

Embracing a Healthier Lifestyle

Changing the way you eat and following a reset plan will help you to embrace a healthier lifestyle. It will involve some change though. Fruits and vegetables contain less calories than say a steak and therefore, you are going to have to eat more to get your energy level stabilized and to also not feel fatigued. You will have to pay attention to your body's needs and add foods that will help you balance out your energy. Specifically, since fruits have a lot of natural sugar, you may need to be more sensitive about your blood sugar levels. Also, when you have an increase in fruit consumption, you might go through some digestive issues. If you add some more vegetables, nuts and low-fiber grains to your diet, you will stabilize your digestive system.

Before the Reset Diet you may have been ruled by your cravings. Do you get up at night to eat something sweet? Does your morning start with a sweet muffin or sugar-laden cereal? If this is the case, you will be happy to know that as you reset your palate, you will lose the desire to eat foods that contain processed sugar.

If you take a bite out of a donut and a bite out of an apple, the donut of course will be sweeter. When you go days without eating that donut, an apple will become a whole lot sweeter to you as your palate for sweet foods will have changed.

Another change that you will be making is to reduce your fat intake. No longer will you eat foods that are processed and high in fat. You will be eating plant-based fats like avocados, olive oil, nuts, seeds and almond milk.

Sometimes there is a concern that you won't be getting the nutrients that you need when you switch to a plant-based diet. True, you might take some supplements. However, if you plan your diet to be high in nutrients you may not need supplements. For example, you can eat dark leafy greens like kale, chard and dandelions and absorb the same amount of calcium as you would get from a cup of milk. Furthermore, vegetables and fruits are high in fiber and have phytonutrients and antioxidants, along with carbohydrates.

How to Start a Reset Diet

So how do you start this Reset Diet? What things can you do to make sure you are successful on the Reset Diet?

The first thing you need for your Reset Diet is to make a

plan. Are you going to ease into the plan or are you going to just jump right in? This is an important thing to figure out. You must reflect on the way you like to do things and match it to the way you are going to handle this reset.

You might just want to start easing off animal proteins and processed foods before you start the Reset Diet plan. You can start with having meatless Mondays and then Tuesdays, etc., or you can just start Day 1 of the plan and get right to it. This is a plan that is flexible for you. It is a plan that builds your confidence instead of tearing it down.

Start the plan by setting a date for when you will start. Be it tomorrow or next week, set the date and make it a hard start date. You might also like to plan your end date. Knowing where you are going to end up is really helpful.

Ways to Make the Reset Diet Easier

The most important thing that you can do for yourself is to commit to doing something that is going to be so very good for you. Develop clear guidelines for yourself about why you are doing a Reset Diet. At first you might want to go on a Reset Diet because you are lacking energy and want to have more energy. As you get more energy from following the Reset Diet, you might even think of other things that you want to accomplish like weight loss. Write down your goals and have a clear picture of how you are going to make them happen while following the Reset Diet. It's always easier to do something if you know exactly why you are doing what you are doing.

THINKING CLEARLY About Your Reset Diet

Another thing to help you on your Reset Diet is for you to set clear directions for yourself. If you tell yourself that you will follow the meal plan as best you can, and if you waver you will allow yourself to skip around the meal plan to find something more appealing. That is a 'rule' that you set for yourself that can help you keep on track. If you make rules for yourself, it will be easier on you when you start to have doubts about what you are doing because you've already decided on a helpful behavior that will lead you to success.

If you make a pledge that you will commit to the reset eating plan, you may find that when times get rough, you are able to stick to the plan. Sometimes it takes more than commitment, it takes accountability. Will you share your goals with someone else? Will you do something definitive like go through your pantry and throw everything out that is toxic to your body?

You may also want to consider other events that are happening in your life. What will be going on in your life as you go on the Reset Diet? Will you be busy? Will it be a peaceful time with no other stressors? Sit down and really think and strategize when will be the best time for you to start the Reset Diet.

Think a little bit more about sharing your goals with someone. Make sure that if you pick a person to help you be accountable, that it is a person that will be supportive and someone who knows how important this is to you. It would be very counterintuitive for you to pick a person who does not believe in your ability to stick to something. Also, a person who doesn't see the benefit of a Reset Diet will also be hard to be around as they won't be supportive. Choose a person who will get excited about your goals and help you to stick to the reset plan. If you can get someone else to go on the Reset Diet with you, excellent!

What to Do After the Reset Plan

Remember that the whole point of the Reset Diet is to gently guide you into following a plant-based diet. Yes, you were focused on the plan ending but what will you do the day after the 'diet' is over? Will you have a juicy hamburger or will you review your reset plan and pick out the meals that worked for you - the meals that you enjoyed the most - and keep eating them. The Reset Diet is a guide for you and a system to follow as you were detoxing and getting your body used to eating plant-based foods. When you finish the Reset Diet, the whole world of plant-based foods will be open to you! You can build on this plan and explore other foods that you might enjoy. Chapter 7 of this book has many recipes for you to explore. There is something for everyone in that chapter. You will find a new world of tastes to enjoy and experiment with.

At the end of the Reset Diet analyze what worked for you. Did you do yoga or any other exercise during the Reset Diet? Was it helpful? Do you now feel healthy enough to start an exercise routine? Did you set-up habits like chopping up all your vegetables when you got home from the grocery store so that it would be easy to grab a snack when you were hungry? What things did you do to make the Reset Diet workable? What habits worked for you and what habits do you need to change?

A Bit About Habits

It's hard to start something and stick with it when you are using only will power. Will power gets you through the first few days but it is going to be practicing healthy and effective habits that will carry you through to the end.

When you make a commitment, you are setting up boundaries for yourself. You have told yourself that you will not eat any animal products or refined sugar. That is a boundary. If you practice habits like preparing your vegetables by chopping them or cooking ahead of time and freezing meals on the weekends, you will find that you depend less and less on will power and more on good habits. The more you stay on track and depend on your habits, the more success you will have in the end. In fact, as you go through the reset plan, depending on your habits, the more your healthy choices will become automatic.

When you are in the thick of the reset plan, remember that you are doing something good for your body. You are eliminating toxins that have been in your body for quite some time. You want to feel better and have the energy to lead a healthier life. You are doing this Reset Diet for yourself but also for the people in your life that love you. When you get better and feel better, you will probably want to share your health with the ones you love. Your loved ones may not be ready for a total change but start slowly to introduce them to what you are learning. Try having a meatless Monday and then increase the meatless days slowly. Become an ambassador for the plant-based diet. Share some of the good food and meals that you have enjoyed. Be confident in your choices and happy with your decisions.

CHAPTER SUMMARY

- The Reset Diet plan is going to add foods that are healing and help with the detox that occurs when you go without the food that was causing you damage. In fact, your metabolism will change due to the fact that you are eating a plant-based diet and not a high calorie dense diet.
- Changing the way you eat and following a reset plan will help you to embrace a healthier lifestyle.
- You will be happy to know that as you reset your palate, you will lose the desire to eat foods that contain processed sugar.
- The first thing you need for your Reset Diet is to make a plan. Are you going to ease into the plan or are you going to just jump right in? This is an important thing to figure out. You must reflect on the way you like to do things and match it to the way you are going to handle this reset.

- When you are in the thick of the reset plan, remember that you are doing something good for your body. You are eliminating toxins that have been in your body for quite some time. You will feel better and have the energy to lead a healthier life.

IN THE NEXT chapter you will learn about the 14-day Detox Plan.

CHAPTER SIX: THE 14-DAY
DETOX PLAN

IN THIS CHAPTER you will learn about the 14-day Detox Plan. I have set out 14 days of breakfast, snack, lunch, dinner and dessert plans for you to ease you into your plant-based diet.

It isn't going to be easy at first, but I have presented you with foods that will give you energy and the nutrients that you will need to nourish you and help your body to get rid of toxins that are in your body.

In the last chapter, we talked about the steps that will help you to stick to this plan. You can do this! The choices that I present can be switched around. If you don't feel like lentil soup on Day 6 but you really liked the spiralized zucchini spaghetti that you had on Day 1, go ahead and switch. The whole object of the 14-day Detox Plan is to fuel your body with the nutrients that your body has been lacking.

Do yourself a favor and find a grocery store that has a big

inventory of the foods that you are going to need. I was very careful to include foods that are commonly available and easy to get. A grocery store that sells tofu, legumes and lots of fresh fruit and vegetables is the one for you.

The 14-day Detox Plan does not require a lot of extreme cooking. You're not going to have to fix some complicated vegan recipes. In fact, you might have fixed this type of meal in your kitchen before. For example, spring salads and taco salads. I also give you a range of smoothie recipes that are sure to please. Plus, they are also easy to put together.

Welcome to the 14-day Detox Plan

I am so excited about your 14-day Detox Plan. There are so many vitamins, antioxidants and lots of nutrients that are going to pull you up and give you lots of energy. Get ready to feel fantastic!

Time is a commodity in our lives. If it's your job or family life that takes the majority of your time, you want a detox plan that is easy to follow. In fact, some of the meals that you will be cooking can be shared with your family or friends who join you at your meals. Black bean burgers might even be more popular than any burger made of beef.

There are also meal ideas that you can buy already made. I provide the recipes for various plant-based desserts but you can also take a short cut and buy these items at your grocery store already made. Some grocery stores may also have pre-made pasta salads that are vegan. Whole wheat rolls, vegan pizza crusts and granola can also be purchased already made.

Don't Fall Into a Trap

The key to buying at the grocery store is for you to read ingredients and make sure that there is no sugar or processed foods in the items that you are going to buy.

Be careful to not fall into the trap of buying vegan convenience foods. For example, you might want to buy vegan burgers that are premade. Read the ingredients and compare them to the recipe that I give you. Be very wary of additives and ingredients that really don't need to be there.

Remember that the goal of the detox plan is to have foods that are whole foods and not procesed foods. The vegan chocolate chip recipe that I am using includes raspberries and the vegan chocolate cake is made from grinding cashews. Look for whole foods when you are shopping for short cuts for the meal plan.

Don't worry, I've kept the recipes really simple. The 14-day Detox Plan is a challenge. It is an adventure to try new tastes and put together foods in a way that you never thought of before. You've had a baked potato before but in this meal plan you don't weigh it done with butter and sour cream. Vegan cheese and vegan bacon crumbles and a side spring salad is a new type of dinner that will get you the nutrients that you need.

If you don't mind eating the same meals within a two-week

period, go ahead and pick out the meals that you like in the detox plan and repeat them as much as you want. If you want to have pizza for lunch more than once, don't hesitate to switch it out with another day. Perhaps you don't care for tofu, so go ahead and have the whole wheat pasta salad instead.

Planning Ahead

This plan is about having easy and practical options, so get ready for the food adventure of your life.

I have designed a practical meal plan so that it is easy to prepare. There are a lot of smoothies in this meal plan. I suggest that you put together the ingredients for the smoothie ahead of time. That way you can put together a smoothie in no time at all because you have prepared. Make a section in your kitchen the smoothie section. Have your ingredients ready to go, already chopped or even frozen.

Planning ahead will really help you to stick to this plan. Organize a shopping list that is easy to use at the grocery store. If you can't find an item in your grocery store, don't be afraid to improvise. If you can't find spiralized zucchini spaghetti but they have another vegetable spiralized spaghetti, by all means, purchase it as a substitute.

There are several salads in this meal plan. I make it easy by using spring mix. Buy a good size bag or container of spring salad for your meal plan. I choose spring salad mix because it keeps a lot better than other salad mixes.

Pick a day to bake and cook some of the recipes that can be made ahead of time. Chop vegetables ahead of time and put them in baggies. Have the snacks in the meal plan ready to eat so that you can have something when you get a craving for a sweet or snack.

In fact, you will have to battle sugar cravings at first, but I have put naturally sweet foods in the plan for you to enjoy. There is a chocolate cake recipe that uses date paste for its sweetness. As you go through the plan and try the smoothies, your palate will be able to enjoy the sweetness of the fruits that you are consuming.

Ways to Make the Detox Plan Easier On You

The 14-day Detox Plan was designed so that you would have a lot of choices. If there is a dish that you don't think you will like, feel free to switch it with something else in the meal plan that you would enjoy.

Each day has a recipe to make but don't be discouraged. The recipes are simple to follow and learn. You can also double the recipe so that you can freeze what you have left over. In fact, you might want to take an afternoon to cook several of the recipes so that you can freeze them. The soups are especially good to make ahead and freeze.

Almost each day there is a smoothie to try. If you find that you have a favorite, repeat that smoothie the next day. It's much easier to assemble the smoothie recipe before hand by cutting up the fruit and putting it in a reusable baggie or container. Then when you want to enjoy the smoothie, you just need to take out the baggie and pour the content into the blender.

The chocolate cake and the cookie in the detox plan can be made ahead and frozen (without the frosting) in individual pieces. The cake may be a bit challenging to make but the taste is well worth the work.

Some of the items in the detox plan can be bought ahead of time. Buy salad mixes that you don't have to chop up. You can even substitute the cake and the cookie recipe for a vegan dessert that is already made. Just be sure that what you are buying is wholesome and does not contain any processed ingredients or an overabundance of sugar. The goal is to get your taste buds back.

Overall, you can make this detox plan as easy as you need it to be. Make the plan your own by rearranging meals. The overall goal is that you adjust to eating whole foods. Good luck. You've got this!

DAY 1

Breakfast: avocado toast, salt, pepper, and slice of whole grain toast

Morning snack: edamame

Lunch: spring mix salad with chickpeas and tomatoes, with whole grain roll

Dinner: spiralized zucchini spaghetti and slice of French bread with garlic and olive oil

Dessert: berry smoothie

Day 2

Breakfast: whole wheat tortilla with tofu scramble with salsa

Snack: trail mix with dried fruit

Lunch: vegetarian chili

Dinner: vegetable kabob

Dessert: vegan peach crisp

Day 3

Breakfast: vanilla blueberry smoothie

Snack: granola with dried fruit

Lunch: taco salad - lettuce, tomatoes, garbanzos and salsa

Dinner: black bean burger with sweet potato fries

Dessert: vegan peanut butter cookies

Day 4

Breakfast: vegan yogurt and granola with dried fruit

Snack: cherry smoothie

Lunch: veggie pizza

Dinner: tofu curry with cauliflower over brown rice, plus spinach salad with olive oil and balsamic vinegar

Dessert: vegan chocolate cake

DAY 5

Breakfast: chia seed pudding with almond milk

Snack: very coconut smoothie

Lunch: whole-wheat pasta salad

Dinner: sweet potato stew

Snack: banana "ice cream" with nut butter (almond, cashew)

DAY 6:

Breakfast: chocolate shake smoothie

Snack: frozen grapes and cantaloupe with 1 ounce of almonds

Lunch: lentil soup with a whole-wheat roll

Dinner: loaded baked potato with vegan cheese and bacon crumbles and side spring salad

Dessert: vegan peanut butter cookies

DAY 7

Breakfast: chia pudding with almond milk and coconut shavings

Snack: roasted chickpeas

Lunch: avocado tacos

Dinner: tofu-stir fry over brown rice

Desert: peach crisp

DAY 8

Breakfast: tofu-scramble with tomato, onion and vegan cheese, plus small bowl of blueberries

Snack: banana slices with cashew butter and raisins

Lunch: tomato soup, French bread and garlic croutons with arugula side salad, chickpeas, fresh tomato, broccoli, red onion, carrots and cucumber with balsamic vinegar and oil.

Dinner: veggie burrito

Dessert: hide the kale smoothie

DAY 9

Breakfast: green smoothie

Snack: granola and vegan yogurt

Lunch: black bean burger on a whole-grain bun with sweet

potato fries

Dinner: tofu curry with roasted vegetables

Dessert: vegan yogurt

DAY 10

Breakfast: mango berry smoothie

Lunch: spring salad mix with roasted peanuts, black beans, cherry tomatoes, strawberries, cucumbers with balsamic dressing

Snack: frozen cantaloupe and honeydew melon balls with handful of almonds

Dinner: lettuce wraps

Dessert: banana 'ice cream' with any nut butter (almond, cashew, etc.)

DAY 11

Breakfast: berry green smoothie

Snack: roasted chickpeas

Lunch: veggie soup

Dinner: portobello mushroom tacos

Desert: vegan peanut butter cookies

DAY 12

Breakfast: avocado goddess smoothie

Snack: chia pudding with almond milk and blueberries

Lunch: Buddha bowl

Snack: hummus and celery sticks

Dinner: spaghetti squash

Dessert: vegan yogurt

DAY 13:

Breakfast: tofu scramble

Snack: steamed edamame with sea salt

Lunch: vegan minestrone soup with spring greens salad with strawberries and balsamic vinaigrette

Dinner: sweet potato stew

DAY 14

Breakfast: vanilla blueberry smoothie

Snack: roasted chickpeas

Lunch: Buddha bowl

Dinner: spaghetti squash

Snack: chia seed pudding with almond milk

*This 14-Day Detox Plan was adapted from a plan on www.eatingwell.com (see citations).

Special Smoothie Recipe Section

Berry Smoothie

Ingredients

- 1 cup frozen blueberries
- 1 cup organic spinach
- 1/2 cup bananas (peeled, sliced, frozen)
- 1 Tbsp flaxseed meal
- 1 1/2 cup orange juice

Directions

1. Put frozen blueberries, bananas and 1 cup of orange juice into the blender.
2. Let blueberries, bananas and orange juice stand for three minutes to thaw.
3. Add the flaxseed meal into the blender and blend for 30 seconds on a low speed.
4. Add the spinach and blend on low for 30 seconds.
5. Add the last half cup of orange juice and blend on high for 1 minute.

6. Pour into glass and enjoy.

If the mixture is too dense, add some more fruit juice or water to break up the dense mixture.

Nutrition (1 of 2 servings)

Serving: 1 smoothie

Calories: 181

Carbohydrates: 41 g

Protein: 2.5 g

Fat: 1.6 g

Vanilla Blueberry Smoothie

Ingredients

- 1/2 cup vegan yogurt
- 1/2 cup cottage cheese
- 1/2 cup frozen blueberries
- 1 tsp vanilla extract
- 2 tsp flaxseed meal
- 1/2 very ripe banana, peeled and frozen
- 10-15 ice cubes
- 1/4 cup water

Directions

1. Put ice cubes and water into the blender and let stand for 1 minute.
2. Add vanilla extract next.
3. Put in the ripe banana and blend on high for 1 minute.
4. Put in cottage cheese, yogurt and blueberry.
5. Blend together on medium for 1 minute.
6. Serve immediately.

Nutrition (1 serving)

Serving: 1 smoothie

Calories: 230

Carbohydrates: 18 g

Protein: 27.5 g

Fat: 5 g

*Nutrition information is a rough estimate.

Notes

- Remember to use vegan cottage cheese or yogurt like soy yogurt.
- You can add a handful of spinach if you want a more nutritious smoothie

PEACH-CHERRY SMOOTHIE

Ingredients

- 1 ripe peach, sliced
- 1 cup frozen cherries
- 3/4 cup soy milk
- 1/4 cup lemon juice
- 1 handful ice
- 1 Tbsp flax seeds
- 1 handful spinach

Directions

1. Add ice and almond milk into the blender and let stand for 1 minute.
2. Add lemon juice.
3. Add peaches and cherries and blend on medium for 1 minute.
4. Add flax seeds and spinach.
5. Blend all ingredients together.
6. Serve immediately.

Note

- You can add more cherries to the smoothie if you want it sweeter.
- You can also freeze this smoothie to be a popsicle.

Nutrition (1 of 2 servings)

Serving: 1 small smoothie

Calories: 150

Carbohydrates: 35 g

Protein: 1.7 g

Fat: 1.3 g

VERY COCONUT SMOOTHIE

Ingredients

- 2 1/4 cups chopped mango
- 1 cup ice
- 1 1/4 cups frozen strawberries
- 1/2 cup crushed pineapple
- 1-2 cups almond milk
- 1/4 cup lemon juice
- 2 Tbsp grated ginger
- 2 Tbsp shredded coconut
- 1/8 teaspoon cayenne pepper
- 1 tsp flax seeds

Directions

1. Add almond milk and ice cubes and let stand for one minute.
2. Add mango, strawberries and pineapple.
3. Add ginger, coconut, cayenne pepper and flax seeds.
4. Blend everything at high speed.
5. Serve immediately.

Nutrition (1 of 2 servings)

Serving: 1 smoothie

Calories: 376

Carbohydrates: 76 g

Protein: 6.6 g

Fat: 10.2 g

Notes

- This smoothie is also good as a popsicle.

CHOCOLATE SHAKE SMOOTHIE

Ingredients

- 2 frozen, very ripe bananas, chopped
- 1/2 cup frozen blueberries
- 3 heaping Tbsp cocoa powder
- 2 Tbsp almond butter
- 1 Tbsp flaxseed meal
- 2 cups soy milk
- 1/3 cup ice
- 1 cup spinach

Directions

1. Add soy milk and ice to the blender and let stand

for 1 minute.

2. Add fruits to the blender and blend on medium for 1 minute.
3. Add cocoa powder, flaxseed and almond butter and blend on medium for 1 minute.
4. Add spinach.
5. Blend at high speed.
6. Serve immediately.

Nutrition (1 of 2 servings)

Serving: 1 smoothie

Calories: 312

Carbohydrates: 48 g

Protein: 6.2 g

Fat: 14 g

BERRY BANANA SMOOTHIE

Ingredients

- 1 medium ripe bananas, frozen
- 1/2 cup frozen blackberries
- 1 heaping Tbsp flax seeds
- 2 cups fresh spinach
- 1 tbsp of almond butter
- 2/3 cup cranberry juice
- 1 1/2 cups water

Directions

1. Add water to the blender.
2. Add cranberry juice.
3. Add fruit and blend on medium for 2 minutes.
4. Add flax seeds, spinach and almond butter.
5. Blend on high for 2 minutes.
6. Serve immediately.

Nutrition (1 of 2 servings)

Serving: 1 smoothie

Calories: 183

Carbohydrates: 37 g

Protein: 3.4 g

Fat: 0.3 g

Green Smoothie

Ingredients

- 1 1/4 cups frozen mango pieces
- 1 cup frozen chunk pineapple
- 1 cup fresh kale
- 1/2 cup water
- 1/2 cup soy milk
- 1 frozen ripe banana

Directions

1. Add water and soy milk to the blender.
2. Add mango and pineapple, blend for a 1 minute.
3. Add ripe banana.
4. Add kale.
5. Blend on high.
6. Serve immediately.

Nutrition (1 of 1 servings)

Serving: 1 smoothie

Calories: 289

Carbohydrates: 65 g

Protein: 6 g

Fat: 3.6 g

Mango Berry Smoothie

Ingredients

- 2 1/4 cups frozen chopped mango
- 1 1/4 cups frozen raspberries
- 1-2 cups soy milk
- 1/4 cup lemon juice
- 3 Tbsp lime juice
- 1 Tbsp freshly grated ginger
- 2 Tbsp unsweetened shredded coconut

- 1 tsp flax seeds
- 1/2 cup of full-fat coconut milk

Directions

1. Add coconut milk and soy milk to the blender.
2. Add ginger and coconut.
3. Blend on medium.
4. Add flax seeds if desired when you serve in a glass.
5. Serve immediately.

Nutrition (1 of 2 servings)

Serving: 1 smoothie

Calories: 376

Carbohydrates: 76 g

Protein: 6.6 g

Fat: 10.2 g

BERRY GREEN SMOOTHIE

Ingredients

- 1 medium frozen banana
- 1/2 cup raspberry berries
- 1 Tbsp chia seeds
- 1 heaping Tbsp natural, salted peanut butter
- 1/2 - 3/4 cup soy milk

- 1 tsp vanilla
- 2 cups fresh spinach

Directions

1. Add vanilla, soy milk to the blender.
2. Add frozen banana and blend for 1 minute.
3. Add chia seeds meal.
4. Add fruit.
5. Add spinach.
6. Blend on high.
7. Serve immediately.

Nutrition

Serving: 1 smoothie

Calories: 314

Carbohydrates: 44.2 g

Protein: 10 g

Fat: 13.4 g

Avocado Goddess Smoothie

Ingredients

- 1 1/2 cup frozen banana
- 1/2 cup crushed pineapple
- 1/2 large ripe avocado

- 1 cup kale
- 1 cup soy milk
- 1/2 cup frozen cucumbers

Directions

1. Add soy milk to the blender.
2. Add frozen banana and cucumbers.
3. Blend on high for 1 minute.
4. Add pineapple, berries and avocado.
5. Blend on high.
6. Serve immediately.

Nutrition (1 of 2 servings)

Serving: 1 smoothie

Calories: 146

Carbohydrates: 18.2 g

Protein: 6.9 g

Fat: 6 g

CHAPTER SEVEN: COOKBOOK

AVOCADO TOAST

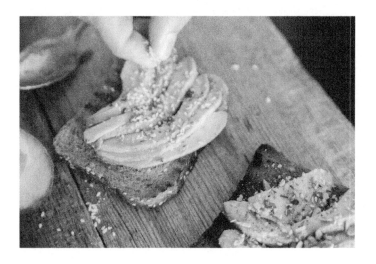

INGREDIENTS

- 1/2 small avocado, sliced or cubed
- 1/2 teaspoon fresh lemon juice
- 1/8 teaspoon kosher salt

- 1/8 teaspoon freshly ground black pepper
- 1 -1 oz slice whole grain bread, toasted
- 1/2 teaspoon extra-virgin olive oil

Directions

1. In a small bowl, combine avocado, lemon juice, salt, and pepper. Gently mash with the back of a fork to soften.
2. Top toasted bread with mashed or sliced avocado mixture.
3. Drizzle with olive oil and sprinkle with desired toppings, such as sesame seeds.

Nutrition

- Calories 200
- Fat 13 g
- Protein 5 g
- Carbohydrates 18 g

Adapted: Cooking Light

AVOCADO TACOS

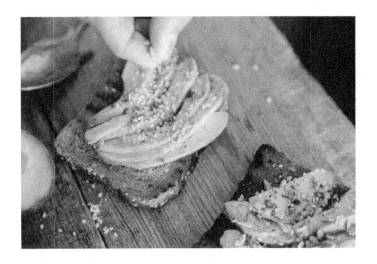

INGREDIENTS

Poblano Ranch Dressing

- 1 poblano chile

- 2 scallions, chopped
- 1/2 cup buttermilk
- 1/4 cup sour cream
- 2 tablespoons fresh lemon juice
- Sea salt, freshly ground pepper

Tacos

- 2 large eggs, beaten to blend
- 1 cup panko or other breadcrumbs
- 1/2 cup all-purpose flour
- 1 avocado, halved, pitted and cut into 8 wedges
- sea salt
- vegetable oil (for frying; about 4 cups)
- 1 15-ounce can refried beans, warmed
- 8 corn tortillas
- 2 cups shredded iceberg lettuce
- 1 cup prepared pico de gallo

Poblano Ranch Dressing

1. Char chile over a gas flame, turning occasionally, until skin is blackened; transfer to a bowl, cover with plastic wrap, and let steam for 15 minutes. Peel, seed, and finely chop.
2. Whisk chile, scallions, buttermilk, sour cream, and lemon juice in a medium bowl.
3. Season with salt and pepper.

Tacos

1. Prepare avocado for frying.
2. Pour egg into a shallow plate or bowl, and pour breadcrumbs in another shallow bowl.
3. Salt avocado wedges.
4. Dredge avocado wedges in flour, then in beaten eggs and then in breadcrumbs. Make sure to shake off excess crumbs.
5. Pour oil into a large deep skillet and heat until the thermometer registers 350°F.
6. Fry avocados in oil until golden (about 3 minutes each).
7. Drain avocados on paper towels to get off excess oil.
8. Heat corn tortillas in the microwave for 1 minute until soft.
9. Spread corn tortillas with warmed beans.
10. Add avocados and then drizzle with Poblano Ranch Dressing.
11. Add lettuce and pico de gallo.

Nutrition

Poblano Dressing

- Calories 46
- Fat 3.3 g
- Carbohydrate 2.7 g
- Protein 1.6 g

Tacos

- Calories 410

- Carbohydrate 58.1g
- Protein 12.2 g

Adapted: bon Appetit

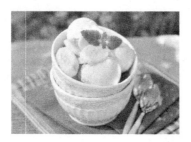

Banana Ice Cream

Servings 1

Ingredients

- Ripe banana

Directions

1. Peel ripe banana and slice into 2" pieces.
2. Put in a plastic zip lock bag and freeze overnight or until solid.
3. Take the banana out of the freezer and place into a blender or food processor.

4. Pulse banana until it is crumbly and scrape down with spatula.
5. Keep pulsing bananas until they are at the gooey stage.
6. Blend banana until it gets smooth and without chunks, scrape down with spatula.
7. Banana will get to a creamy stage.
8. Banana is ready to go back into an airtight container and freeze until it is solid.
9. You can eat it now or wait until it is frozen.
10. The banana should have the texture of ice cream.

Nutrition

- Calories 153
- Fat 9 g
- Carbohydrates 10 g
- Protein 9 g

ADAPTED: thekitchen.com

BLACK BEAN BURGERS

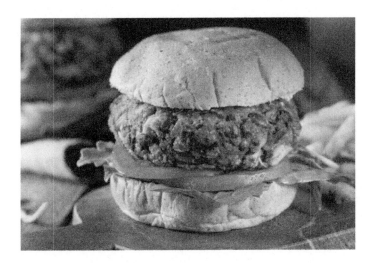

Servings: 4

Ingredients

- 2 Tbsp ground flaxseed

- 3 Tbsp water
- 2-14.5 oz cans black beans, drained and rinsed
- 1 cup panko or other breadcrumbs
- 2 tsp onion powder
- 1 tsp garlic powder
- 2 tsp cumin
- 2 tsp chili powder
- 1 tsp smoked paprika
- 1/2 tsp cayenne pepper
- 1/2 tsp kosher salt
- 1/2 tsp ground black pepper
- Oil/cooking spray, for cooking

Directions

1. Place flax and water in a small bowl. Set aside to thicken.
2. Place beans in a large bowl and mash with potato masher or fork until you have broken up the beans.
3. Add breadcrumbs, onion powder, cumin, chili powder, garlic powder, smoked paprika, cayenne pepper and salt to taste.
4. Add flax mixture and stir until all ingredients are combined.
5. Form 5 bean patties and place in the refrigerator for them to firm up.
6. Spray a large skillet with olive oil and place over medium-high heat.
7. Place patties into the large skillet and cook 10-12 minutes per side or until golden brown.
8. Serve on a bun with desired toppings.

Nutrition

- Calories 439
- Fat 3.1 g
- Carbohydrates 80.1 g
- Protein 24.9 g

Adapted: hummusapian.com

BUDDHA BOWLS

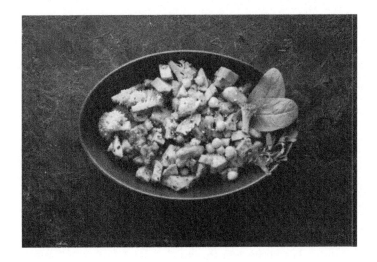

Servings: 6

Ingredients

Vegetables

- 2 Tbsp melted coconut oil
- 1/2 medium red onion, sliced in wedges
- 2 small sweet potatoes, halved
- 1 bundle broccoli chopped and with large stems removed
- 2 big handfuls kale with large stems removed
- 1/4 tsp each of salt and pepper

Chickpeas

- 1 15-ounce chickpeas, drained, rinsed and patted dry
- 1 tsp cumin
- 3/4 tsp chili powder
- 3/4 tsp garlic powder
- 1/4 tsp each salt and pepper
- 1/2 tsp oregano (optional)
- 1/4 tsp turmeric (optional)

Tahini Sauce

- 1/4 cup tahini
- 1 tsp vegan sugar
- 1/2 medium lemon, juiced
- 2-4 Tbsp hot water (to thin)

Directions

1. Preheat the oven to 400°F (204°C) and arrange sweet potatoes and onions on a bare baking sheet.

2. Coat sweet potatoes with melted coconut oil.
3. Bake for 10 minutes, then remove from the oven, flip sweet potatoes and add broccoli.
4. Season with salt and pepper to taste.
5. Bake for another 8-10 minutes, then remove from the oven and add kale.
6. Drizzle kale with oil and season with a pinch each salt and pepper.
7. Bake for another 4-5 minutes then set aside.
8. Mix together spices for chickpeas.
9. Toss chickpeas in spices.
10. Heat oil in a large skillet over-medium heat. Add chickpeas to the skillet.
11. Cook until chickpeas are brown and fragrant. Remove from heat.

Sauce

1. Prepare sauce by adding tahini, vegan sugar and lemon juice to a mixing bowl and whisking together.
2. Add hot water until a pourable sauce is formed. Set aside.
3. Divide sweet potatoes and vegetables into three bowls.
4. Top with chickpea mixture.
5. Drizzle tahini dressing over the three bowls.

Nutrition

- Calories 388
- Fat 12.8 g
- Carbohydrates 54.8 g
- Protein 17.3 g

Adapted: minimalistbaker.com

CHIA PUDDING

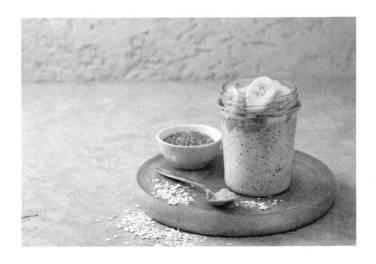

Serving: 1 bowl or jar

Ingredients

- 2 Tbsp chia seeds

- 1/2 cup almond milk
- 1 tsp any natural sweetener of your choice
- Any berry for garnishing

Directions

1. Add ingredients into a mason jar and shake vigorously to mix together chia seeds with milk.
2. Cover the jar and place in the fridge for 2-3 hours or overnight.
3. The mixture is done when it looks like tapioca.
4. Serve immediately and garnish with berries of your choice.

Nutrition

- Calories 155
- Fat 8 g
- Carbohydrates 16 g
- Protein 4 g

Adapted: feelgoodfoodie.net

CHOCOLATE CAKE

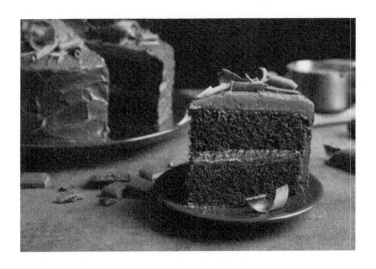

Ingredients

Cake

- 2 cups whole wheat flour

- 1 tsp baking powder
- 1 tsp baking soda
- 1/2 tsp sea salt
- 1/2 cup unsweetened cocoa powder
- 1 cup date paste (3/4 cup unrefined sugar for those not doing sugar-free)
- 3/4 cup applesauce
- 1 1/4 cup almond milk
- 2 tsp vanilla
- 1 Tbsp apple cider vinegar

Frosting

- 1 cup cooked sweet potato, peeled
- 1/2 cup almond or cashew butter
- 3/4 cup dates, pitted (3/4 cup unrefined sugar for those not doing sugar-free)
- 1/4 cup almond milk
- 1/2 cup cocoa powder
- 1/4 tsp sea salt
- 1 Tbsp vanilla

Directions

Cake

1. Preheat the oven to 350°F.
2. Prepare two 8x8 baking pans with non-stick spray.
3. Make date paste by mixing date paste with 3/4 cup water and blend in the food processor. Set aside.

4. Whisk together baking powder, baking soda, cocoa powder in a large bowl.
5. In another large bowl mix together applesauce, almond milk, vanilla, vinegar and date paste. Mix together well.
6. Mix dry ingredients into wet ingredients.
7. Pour mixture into prepared baking pans.
8. Bake for 30 minutes.
9. Remove from the oven and let cool before frosting.

Frosting

1. Poke holes in the sweet potato with a fork. Place in the microwave for 5 minute to cook. Adjust cooking time according to the size of sweet potato.
2. Mash sweet potato and put it in a food processor bowl along with other frosting ingredients.
3. Process mixture until smooth.
4. Frost cake with frosting when cake is cool.

Nutrition

- Calories 341
- Carbohydrates 72.3 g
- Protein 7.4 g

Adapted: eatplantbased.com

CRANBERRY CRISP

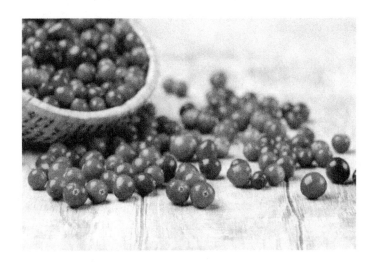

Servings: 8

Ingredients

- 2 Tbsp cornstarch

- Two 16-oz. pkg. frozen unsweetened peach slices, thawed, or 6 cups sliced fresh peaches
- 1 cup fresh or frozen cranberries
- 1 cup whole wheat pastry flour
- 1/2 cup rolled oats
- 1/4 cup vegan sugar
- 1 tablespoon chia seeds
- 1 1/2 teaspoons baking powder
- 1/2 teaspoon ground cinnamon
- 1/2 cup unsweetened almond milk
- 1/4 cup unsweetened applesauce
- 1/4 cup cashew butter

Directions

1. Preheat the oven to 400°F.
2. In a large Dutch oven combine the 1/4 cup sugar, the cornstarch, and 1/4 cup water.
3. Add peaches to the mixture in the Dutch oven. Cook and stir over medium until slightly thick and bubbly.
4. Stir in cranberries. Transfer hot mixture to a 2-qt. baking dish.

For Topping

1. In a medium bowl stir together whole wheat pastry four, rolled oats, sugar, chia seeds, baking powder, and cinnamon.

2. Whisk together in a separate bowl, milk, applesauce, and cashew butter.
3. Add milk mixture to flour mixture and stir to combine everything.
4. Add the combined flour mixture to the fruit mixture in the baking dish. You can use a spoon to drop mixture onto fruit mixture.
5. Bake for 25 minutes, until golden brown and bubbly.

Nutrition

- Calories 217
- Fat 3.1 g
- Carbohydrate 45.4 g
- Protein 4 g

Adapted: forksoverknifes.com

EVERYDAY VEGAN LENTIL SOUP

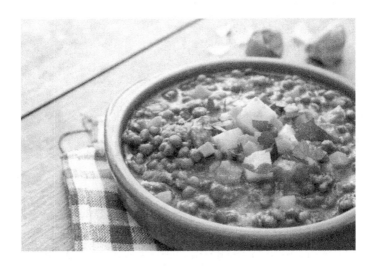

Servings: 8

Ingredients

- 2 Tbsp olive oil

- 1 medium white onion, chopped
- 3 cloves garlic, minced
- 2 medium carrots, peeled and chopped
- 2 celery ribs, diced
- 14-ounce can diced tomatoes
- 2 cups dry brown lentils
- 7 cups vegetable broth
- 1/2 tsp ground cumin
- 1/2 tsp ground coriander
- 1 tsp smoked paprika
- 1/2 tsp cayenne (optional)
- 1 tsp salt, or to taste
- 2 cups spinach, sliced into ribbons
- 1 cup kale
- 1 lemon, juiced (about 2 Tbsp)

Directions

1. Heat the olive oil in a large Dutch oven, over medium heat. Add the onions, garlic, carrots, and celery. Stir frequently for 5 minutes.
2. Add spices and stir for 1 minute.
3. Now add the can of tomatoes (with juices), lentils and vegetable broth. Stir to incorporate everything.
4. Bring to a boil, then lower heat to a simmer and cook for about 30 minutes, until the lentils are tender and the soup has thickened.
5. Stir in the spinach and lemon juice and let the spinach wilt.
6. Season with salt to taste.

Nutrition

- Calories 152
- Fat 5 g
- Carbohydrates 17.9 g
- Protein 10 g

Adapted: noracooks.com

GRANOLA

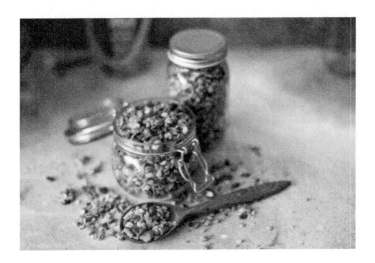

Ingredients

- 2 cups rolled oats. If you have a gluten sensitivity use gluten free oats.
- 1/2 cup raw pecans chopped

- 1/4 cup pumpkin seeds
- 1/4 cup almond butter
- 1/2 tsp vanilla extract
- 2 tbsp chia seeds
- 1/4 cup dried sugar-free cranberries

Directions

1. Preheat the oven to 300°F.
2. Spray cookie sheet with non-stick spray.
3. In a large bow, mix together oats, chopped nuts, pumpkin seeds, chia seeds, and cranberries.
4. Stir in almond butter and vanilla extract over oat mixture. Combine well.
5. Pour mixture onto cookie sheet.
6. Place into the oven and bake for 9 minutes (be careful not to burn the mixture).
7. Take out of the oven and cool completely.

Nutrition

- Calories 223
- Fat 11.9 g
- Carbohydrates 25 g
- Protein 6.1 g

Adapted: Keepingthepeas.com

HEALTHY VEGAN LETTUCE WRAPS

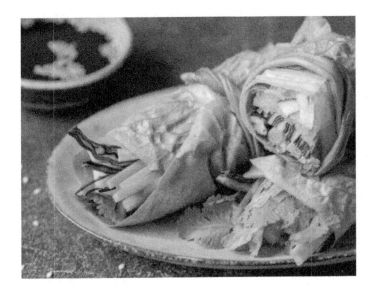

Ingredients

- 1 Tbsp olive oil
- 1 medium white onion chopped

- 1 orange bell pepper chopped
- 3 cloves garlic, minced or pressed
- 1 Tbsp ginger paste
- 8 ounces tempeh
- 2 Tbsp soy sauce
- 1 lime, juiced
- 3 green onions sliced
- 8-10 butter lettuce leaves
- 1 cup shredded or julienned carrots
- 1 cup shredded red cabbage
- 1/2 cup chopped peanuts
- 1/4 cup fresh cilantro roughly or finely chopped
- Sriracha sauce

Directions

1. Heat oil in a nonstick skillet over medium-high heat.
2. Add onion, bell pepper, and cook until the onion is translucent and the bell pepper is soft.
3. Add ginger past and cook for 20 seconds.
4. Add garlic and stir for 20 seconds.
5. Add the tempeh and cook for 5 minutes or until lightly browned.
6. Add lime juice, soy sauce and green onions.
7. Take the mixture off the heat and let cool slightly.
8. Prepare the lettuce leaves.
9. Spoon tempeh mixture into middle of lettuce leaves.
10. Add 1/4 cup carrots, red cabbage to lettuce leaf.
11. Sprinkle 1 Tbsp of peanuts over the mixture.
12. Add cilantro and Sriracha sauce to taste.

13. Wrap up lettuce leaf like a burrito.

Nutrition

- Calories 153
- Fat 9 g
- Carbohydrates 10 g
- Protein 9 g

PEACH CRISP

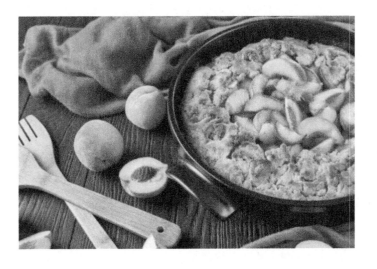

Servings: 4

Ingredients

- 1/3 cup whole rolled oats
- 1/3 cup chopped pecans
- 1/4 cup all-purpose flour
- 1/2 teaspoon cinnamon
- pinch of salt
- 3 Tbsp hardened coconut oil (plus more for the skillet)
- 4 peaches, sliced
- 4 plums, sliced

Directions

1. Preheat the oven to 350°F .
2. Prepare an 8x8 baking dish with coconut oil.
3. Add oats, pecans, flour, sugar, cinnamon and salt to the food processor and pulse until mixture is crumbly. Add a little bit of water if the mixture is too dry. Be careful not to make it too wet. If this happens add a little more flour until you get desired moistness.
4. Put fruit slices into the pan and cover with flour mixture.
5. Bake for 15 minutes until the mixture is golden brown.
6. Let cool and then serve.

Nutrition

- Calories 295

- Fat 13.2 g
- Carbohydrates 44 g
- Protein 3.9 g

Adapted: loveandlemons.com

VEGAN PEANUT BUTTER COOKIES

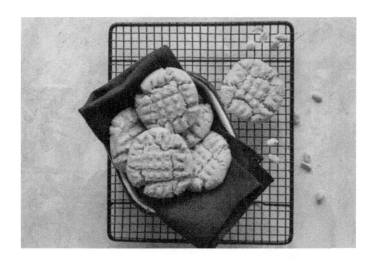

Dry Ingredients

- 1 cup oat flour
- 1/2 tsp baking powder
- 1/2 tsp baking soda

- 1/4 tsp salt

Wet Ingredients

- 3/4 cup natural, unsalted creamy peanut butter
- 3 Tbsp melted coconut oil
- 1/2 cup coconut sugar
- 1 very ripe banana mashed, for sweetness (optional)
- 2 flax 'eggs' (whisk together 2 Tbsp ground flax and 6 Tbsp warm water and let set for 15 minutes)
- 1 tsp pure vanilla extract

Directions

1. Preheat the oven to 350°F.
2. Prepare the baking sheet with non-stick spray.
3. In a large bowl whisk together oat flour, baking powder and salt.
4. In a medium bowl, mix together the peanut butter, mashed banana, oil, sugar, flax 'eggs' and vanilla.
5. Mix together wet ingredients with dry ingredients.
6. Use a cookie scooper to drop cookies onto the prepared baking sheet. Cookie dough will be hard to work with since it is very sticky, so take your time.
7. When cookie dough is on the baking sheet, use a fork to flatten cookies. Use a fork to make the traditional peanut butter cookie criss cross decoration.
8. Bake for 10-14 minutes.

9. Take cookies out and let cool slightly in pans.
10. When cookies are more solid, remove from the tray and finish cooling on a wire rack.

Nutrition

- Calories 202
- Fat 15 g
- Carbohydrates 12 g
- Protein 6 g

Adapted: Beamingbaker.com

VEGGIE PIZZA

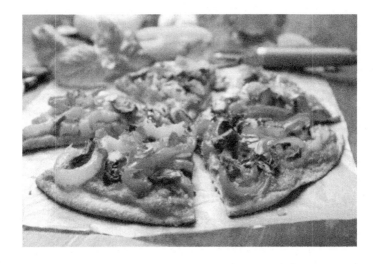

Ingredients

Pizza Dough

- 1 cup warm water
- 1 packet fast-acting yeast
- 2 cups all-purpose flour
- 2 Tbsp olive oil (+ more for seasoning crust)
- 2 Tbsp sugar, divided
- 1 tsp salt (and a bit more for crust)
- 1/2 tsp garlic powder
- 1 tsp powdered milk
- shortening for pizza pan

Toppings

- 1/2 cup store bought pizza sauce
- vegan mozzarella cheese, shredded
- 1/2 cup fresh basil, chopped
- 1 small white onion sliced
- 1/2 cup red bell pepper, diced
- any roasted vegetable of your choice

Directions

Pizza Dough

1. Preheat the oven to 500°F.
2. Stir yeast and 1/2 Tbsp sugar into warmed water until dissolved. Let it sit for 7-10 minutes, until foamy.
3. Add flour, garlic powder, salt, and remaining sugar into a large bowl. Whisk together ingredients until combined.

4. Add the yeast mixture to the bowl along with olive oil.

5. Mixed together ingredients until dough forms a ball.

6. Place in an oiled bowl and cover with a clean kitchen towel. Leave the dough to rise for about 30 minutes or until the dough doubles.

7. Prepare the pizza pan by lightly spreading the shortening onto the pan.

8. When dough is ready spread out onto the pan - use fingers to take dough to the edge of the pan.

Toppings

1. Add store bought sauce to the pizza crust using a spoon to spread it onto the edges.

2. Sprinkle shredded mozzarella over the pizza.

3. Distribute basil, red bell pepper and onion evenly over pizza.

4. Add any vegetable toppings you like.

5. Bake for 10-15 minutes, until the crust is golden brown. The pizza cooks fast so keep an eye on it.

Nutrition

- Calories 189
- Fat 3 g
- Carbohydrates 32 g
- Protein 3 g

Notes

* Makes 2 10-inch pizzas.

* Nutritional info does not contain the mozzarella cheese topping.

PORTOBELLO MUSHROOM TACOS

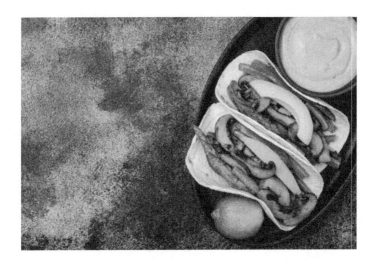

Servings: 2

Ingredients

Taco

- 2 extra-large portobello mushrooms
- 1 green bell pepper
- 1/2 white onion (optional)

Chipotle Marinade

- 1 Tbsp olive oil
- 2 Tbsp canned chipotle in adobo sauce
- 1 minced garlic clove or a 1/2 teaspoon granulated garlic
- 1/2 tsp cumin
- 1/2 tsp coriander
- salt to taste
- 4 tortillas, warmed
- 1 can refried black beans, warmed
- optional toppings
- avocado
- pico de gallo

Directions

1. Preheat the oven to 425°F.
2. Prepare mushrooms by cutting into 1/2-inch-thick wedges, slice bell pepper into strips and cut onion into rings.
3. Place mushrooms, bell peppers and onion on a jelly roll pan.

Marinade

1. Combine oil, garlic, and spices to make marinate. Whisk ingredients together.
2. Brush vegetables with marinade and leave for ten minutes.
3. Sprinkle vegetables with salt.
4. Put the vegetables into the oven and roast for 20 minutes.
5. Heat tortillas in the microwave for 1 minute or until soft.
6. Spread tortillas with warm refried beans.
7. Take out vegetables and let cool for 5 minutes.
8. Add vegetables to tacos and serve immediately.

Nutrition

Tacos

- Calories 50
- Fat 0.2 g
- Carbohydrates 10.1 g
- Protein 3.9 g

Adapted: feastingathome.com

TOFU CURRY WITH CAULIFLOWER

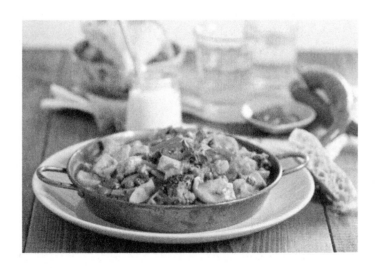

Servings: 8

Ingredients

- 1 Tbsp olive oil

- 1 carrot, sliced
- 1 small white onion, chopped
- 3 tsp curry powder
- 1/4 tsp salt
- 1/4 tsp pepper
- 1 small head cauliflower, broken into florets (about 3 cups)
- 1 can (14-1/2 ounce) diced tomatoes
- 1 package (14 ounces) extra-firm tofu, drained and cut into 1/2-inch cubes
- 1 cup vegetable broth
- 1 can (15 ounces) chickpeas, rinsed and drained
- 1 can (14 ounces) coconut milk
- 1 cup frozen peas
- hot cooked rice
- chopped fresh cilantro

Directions

1. In a medium stockpot, heat oil over medium-high heat. Add carrots and onion; cook and stir until onion is tender, 5 minutes.
2. Stir in curry powder, salt, and pepper.
3. Add cauliflower, tomatoes, tofu, and broth to the stockpot and bring to a boil. Reduce heat, simmer covered for 12 minutes.
4. Add chickpeas, coconut milk and peas and return to a boil. Reduce heat to medium. Cook uncovered, stirring occasionally for 5-7 minutes.
5. Serve immediately over rice. Sprinkle with cilantro.

Nutrition

- Calories 411
- Fat 19.8 g
- Carbohydrates 44.6 g
- Protein 19.2 g

Adapted: tasteofhome.com

TOFU SCRAMBLE

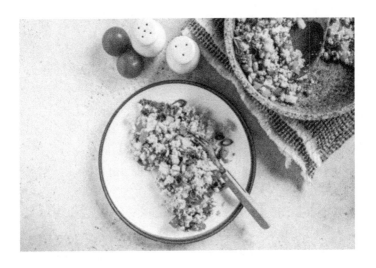

Serving: 1

Ingredients

- 8 ounces extra-firm tofu

- 1-2 Tbsp olive oil
- 1/4 red onion (thinly sliced)
- 1/2 red pepper (thinly sliced)
- 2 cups kale (loosely chopped)
- Sauce
- 1/2 tsp sea salt (reduce amount for less salty sauce)
- 1/2 tsp garlic powder
- 1/2 tsp ground cumin
- 1/4 tsp chili powder
- Water (to thin)
- 1/4 tsp turmeric (optional)

Directions

1. Dry tofu gently to wipe away moisture. Lay something heavy on top of it to flatten and let drain for 15 minutes.
2. Prepare spices in a small bowl. Add water to make a paste.
3. In a medium skillet over medium-high heat, add olive oil, onion, red pepper and salt and pepper (optional).
4. Cook onion and red peppers until soft.
5. While tofu is draining, prepare sauce by adding dry spices to a small bowl and adding enough water to make a pourable sauce. Set aside.
6. Place kale in a skillet and cover for 2 minutes.
7. Use a fork to crumble tofu into small pieces.
8. Remove vegetables from the skillet and add tofu. Stir-fry for 2 minutes and then add spice paste and cook for 5-7 minutes until tofu is browned.

9. Add vegetables back into the skillet and cook together for 1 minute.
10. Add kale, season with a bit more salt and pepper, and cover to steam for 2 minutes.
11. In the meantime, unwrap tofu and use a fork to crumble into bite-sized pieces.
12. Take off the cover on the skillet and remove vegetables.
13. Add tofu to skillet and cook until browned.
14. Add vegetables back in and cook together for 1 minute.
15. Serve immediately.

Nutrition

- Calories 212
- Carbohydrates 7.1 g
- Protein 16.4 g
- Fat 15.1 g

Adapted: minimalistbaker.com

TOFU AND VEGETABLE SKEWERS

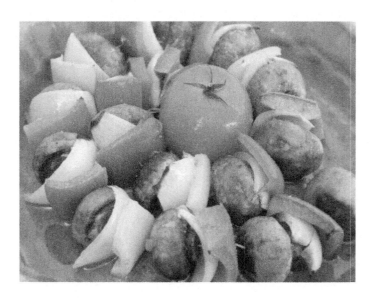

Ingredients

- 8 ounce container extra firm tofu, drained and
  sliced into large chunks

- 1 zucchini, cut into large chunks
- 1 red bell pepper, cut into large chunks
- 10 large mushrooms
- 2 tablespoons sriracha chili garlic sauce
- 1/4 cup soy sauce
- 2 tablespoons sesame oil
- 1/4 cup diced onion
- 2 jalapeno peppers, diced
- 1 pinch ground black pepper to taste

Directions

1. In a small bowl mix together sriracha sauce, soy sauce, sesame oil, onion, jalapenos and pepper. Mix together.
2. Assemble tofu, red bell pepper, mushrooms, zucchini in a bowl and pour sauce over vegetables and toss to cover completely.
3. Cover bowl and place in refrigerator to marinate for 1 hour or overnight.
4. After vegetables are marinated, take them out of the refrigerator.
5. Place vegetables on a skewer in desired order.
6. Preheat an outdoor or indoor grill to medium-high heat, and lightly oil the grate.
7. When the grill is ready, place skewers on the grill and cook for 10 minutes until done to your desired softness.

Nutrition

- Calories 301
- Fat 19.8 g
- Carbohydrates 19.4 g
- Fat 19.8 g

Adapted: allrecipes.com

TOFU STIR FRY

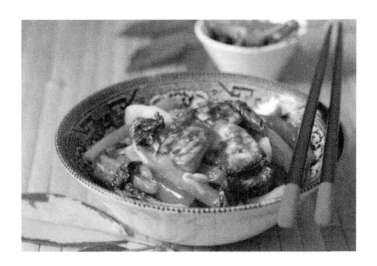

Ingredients

- 2 x 14-ounce packages extra-firm tofu. Do not use firm, silken or anything other than extra-firm
- 1 Tbsp canola oil

- 3 Tbsp soy sauce - divided, plus additional to taste
- 3 large garlic cloves - minced, about 1 heaping Tbsp
- 1 small bunch green onions - finely chopped, divided
- 1 Tbsp minced fresh ginger
- 1/4-1/2 tsp red pepper flakes
- 10 ounces baby spinach
- 2 Tbsp sesame oil

For Serving

- Prepared brown rice or Quinoa

Directions

1. Drain the tofu. Wrap each block in a double layer of paper towels and pat dry, pressing down on the tofu lightly to squeeze out excess moisture. Cut the tofu into 3/4-inch cubes.
2. In a large nonstick wok or frying pan, heat the oil over medium high heat.
3. Add tofu and drizzle soy sauce over it. Sauté until the tofu is browned on each side and moisture is cooked out of it - about 8-10 minutes.
4. Add the garlic, roughly two-thirds of the green onion, ginger, red pepper flakes and the remaining 2 Tbsp soy sauce. Mix everything together and let cook for 1 minute.
5. Add several large handfuls of spinach and stir gently

until the spinach wilts. Keep adding spinach and cooking until the whole batch is done.

6. Stir in the sesame oil and remove from heat.
7. Add the rest of the green onions and serve over brown rice.
8. Add more red pepper flakes and soy sauce to taste.
9. Remove from the heat. Sprinkle the reserved green onions over the top.
10. Serve hot, with brown rice, noodles, or whatever you like, along with a few dashes of additional soy sauce and chili paste or flakes to taste.

Nutrition

- Calories 297
- Fat 17 g
- Carbohydrates 12 g
- Protein 22 g

Adapted: wellplated.com

TOFU BREAKFAST SCRAMBLE

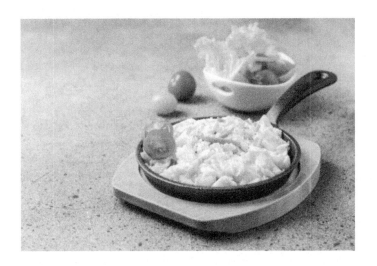

Serving: 1

Ingredients

- 1 Tbsp olive oil
- 1 x 16-ounce block firm tofu
- 2 Tbsp nutritional yeast
- 1/2 tsp salt, or more to taste
- 1/4 tsp turmeric
- 1/4 tsp garlic powder
- 2 Tbsp almond milk

For Garnish

- Avocado sliced into wedges and cilantro
- Cherry tomatoes

Directions

1. Heat olive oil in a pan over medium-high heat.
2. Crumble the tofu and add it to the pan and cook for 4 minutes until the moisture from the tofu has evaporated.
3. Add the nutritional yeast, salt, turmeric, and garlic powder to the scramble and cook for five minutes.
4. Add milk to the mixture and stir to mix.
5. Serve immediately.
6. Garnish with avocado and cilantro.

Nutrition

- Calories 288
- Fat 18 g

- Carbohydrates 9 g
- Protein 24 g

Adapted: noracooks.com

HOMEMADE TOMATO SOUP

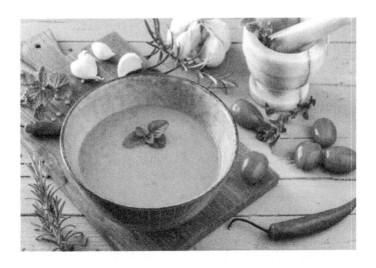

Servings: 2

Ingredients

- 2 Tbsp olive oil
- 1 medium yellow onion, chopped
- 4 garlic cloves, minced
- 28 ounces canned diced tomatoes
- 1/2 cup of basil, chopped
- 2 cups vegetable broth
- 1/2 cup almond milk
- 1/2 tsp salt, or more to taste
- 1 tsp granulated sugar, optional to cut the acidity

Directions

1. In a large pot heat the olive oil over medium-high heat.
2. Add the chopped onion and stir-fry for 5 minutes or until the onion and garlic is translucent. Be careful not to burn the garlic.
3. Add the diced tomatoes, basil and vegetable broth and stir together. Bring to a boil and then turn down and simmer for 15 minutes.
4. Add almond milk. You can leave it out if you don't want the soup to be creamy.
5. Stir in sugar to cut the acidity of the soup if you like.
6. Blend soup in a blender if you would like a smoother soup.
7. Serve immediately.

Nutrition

- Calories 173
- Fat 8 g
- Carbohydrates 25 g
- Protein 6 g

Adapted: noracooks.com

TACO SALAD

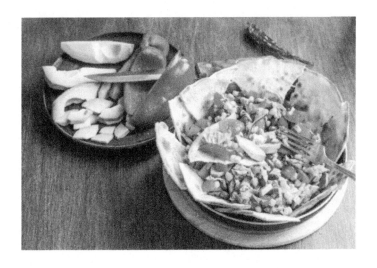

Ingredients

Black Beans

- 1 15-ounce can black beans, rinsed and drained, or 1 1/2 cups cooked black beans
- 2 tsp chili powder
- 1/4 tsp cayenne pepper
- 1/2 tsp salt
- 1/2 tsp garlic powder
- 1/2 tsp smoked paprika
- 1 tsp cumin
- 1/4 cup water

Crunchy Roasted Chickpeas

- 1 15-ounce can chickpeas, rinsed, drained, and dried really well, or 1 1/2 cups cooked chickpeas
- 1 tsp chili powder
- 1 tsp cumin
- 1/2 tsp cayenne pepper
- 1/2 tsp salt

Salad

- 1 head iceberg lettuce, chopped
- 1-cup cherry tomatoes, halved
- 1/2 cup red bell pepper, diced
- 1/2 cup green bell pepper
- 2 small avocados, diced

Dressing

- 1 recipe Southwest Vegan Ranch Dressing

- 3/4 cup raw cashews, soaked for 1 to 2 hours if you don't have a high-speed blender
- 1/2 cup water
- juice of 1 lemon, about 2 Tbsp
- 1 Tbsp apple cider vinegar
- 1 clove garlic
- 1/2 tsp onion powder
- 1 tsp dried dill
- 1 tsp snipped chives
- 1/2 tsp dried oregano
- 1/2 tsp salt, (or to taste)
- 1 tsp cumin
- 1/2 tsp smoked paprika

Directions for Dressing

1. Blend all ingredients in a high-speed blender until smooth. Add additional water by the tablespoon if needed to thin.

Directions for Chickpeas

1. Preheat the oven to 400°F.
2. Toss chickpeas with the chili powder, cumin, salt and cayenne.
3. Place chickpeas on a jelly roll sheet pan in one even layer and bake for 20 to 30 minutes.
4. When chickpeas are golden and crunchy, take them out of the oven to cool. Set aside.
5. In a pan over medium heat, add black beans and

then spices, add 1/4 cup water to the pan and mix everything together, cook until warmed through.

6. Assemble salad and then toss with dressing.
7. Serve on individual plates and add black bean mixture and chickpeas.

Nutrition

Dressing

- Calories 149
- Fat 11.9 g
- Carbohydrates 8.7 g
- Protein 4 g

Salad

- Calories 454
- Fat 21.5 g
- Carbohydrates 56.8 g
- Protein 13.8 g

Adapted: veggieinspired.com

ROASTED CHICKPEAS

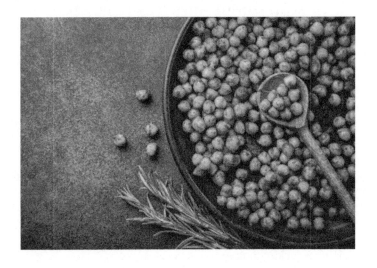

Servings: 8 (makes about 2 cups)

Ingredients

- 2 x 15-ounce cans chickpeas

- 2 Tbsp olive oil
- 1 to 1 1/2 tsp sea salt
- 2 to 4 tsp chili powder

Directions

1. Heat the oven to 400°F. Arrange a rack in the middle of the oven.
2. Rinse and drain chickpeas and then pat dry.
3. Pour chickpeas onto a jelly roll pan.
4. Toss chickpeas with olive oil, salt, and chili powder until well coated.
5. Place chickpeas in the oven and cook until golden brown or 20-30 minutes. Stir the chickpeas midway and be careful not to let them burn.

Nutrition

- Calories 417
- Fat 9.9 g
- Carbohydrates 64.5 g
- Protein 20.5 g

Adapted: thekitchn.com

SPAGHETTI SQUASH W/ CHICKPEAS & KALE

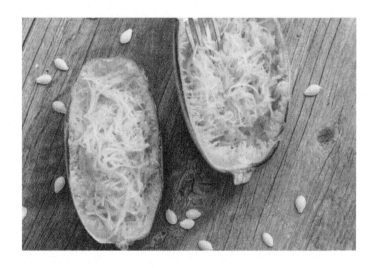

Servings: 4

Ingredients

- 1 spaghetti squash

- 1-2 Tbsp olive oil
- 1 whole garlic clove
- 1/2 Tbsp minced fresh rosemary
- 1/4 tsp of chile flakes
- 1/2 cup chickpeas, cooked drained and rinsed
- 2 (packed) cups chopped kale leaves
- 1 Tbsp lemon juice
- 1/4 cup chopped black olives
- 1/4 cup toasted pine nuts
- kosher salt and freshly ground black pepper

Directions

1. Preheat the oven to 400°F.
2. Cut spaghetti squash in half.
3. Remove the seeds.
4. Place spaghetti squash on a baking sheet and bake for 40 minutes.
5. Take out spaghetti squash and let cool for ten minutes.
6. Shred spaghetti squash with a fork to get the spaghetti strands and put aside.
7. In a nonstick skillet over medium heat, add olive oil.
8. Add garlic, rosemary, chili flakes and salt and pepper and cook for 3 minutes careful not to burn garlic.
9. Add chickpeas and cook for 3 minutes or until chickpeas turn a golden brown.
10. Remove garlic from skillet and add the kale, the chopped olives and salt and pepper to taste.

11. Add the spaghetti strands from squash and mix everything together.
12. Remove from heat and add toasted pine nuts.
13. Serve immediately.

Nutrition

- Calories 248
- Fat 14.5 g
- Carbohydrates 25.3 g
- Protein 7.8 g

Adapted: loveandlemons.com

SWEET POTATO FRIES

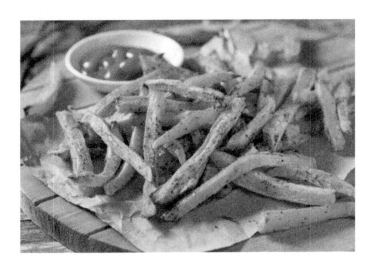

Ingredients

- 2 pounds sweet potatoes, peeled and cut into sticks 1/4 wide and 1/4-inch-thick (about 2 medium-large or 3 medium)

- 1 Tbsp cornstarch
- 1/2 tsp salt
- 2 Tbsp virgin olive oil
- optional spices: freshly ground black pepper, cayenne pepper and/or garlic powder

Directions

1. Preheat the oven to 425°F.
2. Spray two jelly roll baking sheets with non-stick cooking spray.
3. Place sweet potato fries onto a jelly roll sheet so that they aren't too crowded.
4. Sprinkle lightly with cornstarch and salt and toss until coated. Make sure there are no clumps.
5. Sprinkle olive oil lightly over the fries and make sure that each one is coated well.
6. Bake fries on one side for twenty minutes and then flip the fries over.
7. Bake for 10-18 minutes longer.
8. Take out fries and sprinkle with 1/4 tsp cayenne pepper and salt to taste.

Nutrition

- Calories 263
- Fat 7.1 g
- Carbohydrates 47.4 g
- Protein 3.6 g

Adapted: cookieandkate.com

SWEET POTATO STEW

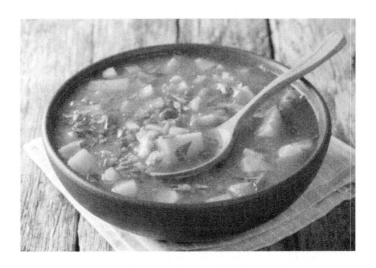

Ingredients

- 2 tsp olive oil
- 2 small yellow onions, diced
- 2 red bell peppers, diced

- 2 green bell peppers, diced
- 4 cloves garlic, minced
- 2 tsp cumin
- 1 tsp turmeric
- 1 tsp ginger
- 2 tsp coriander
- 1/2 tsp cinnamon
- 1 tsp red pepper flakes (optional)
- 4 cups vegetable broth
- 6 cups, peeled and diced sweet potato
- 2 -28 oz cans diced tomatoes with their juices
- 2 -19 oz can chickpeas, rinsed and drained
- 1/2 cup natural peanut butter
- 1/2 cup raisins, chopped roughly
- 1 cup finely chopped cilantro, about 40 g
- 2 tbsp fresh lemon juice
- salt and black or white pepper, to taste

Directions

1. In a soup pot over medium heat olive oil and then sauté onion and garlic until onion is translucent. Be careful not to burn garlic.
2. Add cumin, turmeric, ginger, coriander, and cinnamon and cook for one minute.
3. Add the bell peppers, diced tomatoes and sweet potato and broth stir to combine and simmer for 15-20 minutes letting the sweet potato get tender.
4. Add chickpeas, raisons, peanut butter and stir until the peanut butter is well mixed with everything in the pot.

5. Add lemon and cilantro and turn off heat and let sit for 5 minutes before serving.

6. Stir in the chickpeas, dates or raisins, peanut butter, lemon, and cilantro. Stir until the peanut butter is completely mixed in. Turn off the heat and let sit for a few minutes to allow everything to heat through.

7. Serve right away topped with fresh cilantro, red pepper flakes and chopped peanuts or cashews, if desired.

8. Leftovers can be stored in the fridge for up to 5 days or frozen for up to 3 months.

Nutrition

- Calories 236
- Fat 6.5 g
- Carbohydrates 36 g
- Protein 9 g

Adapted: runingonrealfood.com

VEGAN BURRITO

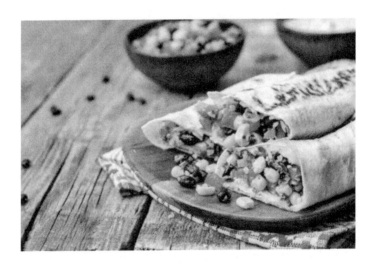

Ingredients

- 1/2 cup cooked rice (white or brown) or quinoa
- 2 Tbsp olive oil or 1/4 cup water
- 1/2 large onion, diced

- 1/2 green bell pepper, cored and diced
- 1 can (4 oz) tomato and diced green chilies, drained
- 1 large jalapeno, diced
- 1/2 tsp cumin
- 1/2 Tbsp chili powder
- 1/2 tsp tsp cayenne
- 1 tsp garlic powder
- 1/2 tsp salt, or to taste
- 1/2 cup sweet corn
- 1 cup black beans, drained and rinsed
- 1/4 cup cilantro, loosely packed
- 2 large flour tortillas, or your favorite gluten-free tortillas
- 1 cup shredded lettuce
- 1/2 cup diced fresh tomato
- guacamole or sliced avocado, optional

Directions

1. Add oil to the saucepan and heat over medium-high heat.
2. Add onion, green bell pepper, and cook until soft.
3. Add spices: cumin, chili powder, cayenne, garlic powder and salt and cook for 1 minute.
4. Add black beans and mash with potato masher, but leave some beans whole.
5. Add corn and heat through.
6. Heat tortilla on a griddle for 2 minutes on each side.
7. Add black bean mixture to the tortilla and wrap like a burrito.

8. Top with lettuce, fresh tomato and diced jalapeno.

Nutrition

- Calories 369
- Fat 9.7 g
- Carbohydrates 60.9 g
- Protein 11.7 g

Adapted: simple-veganista.com

VEGAN CHILI

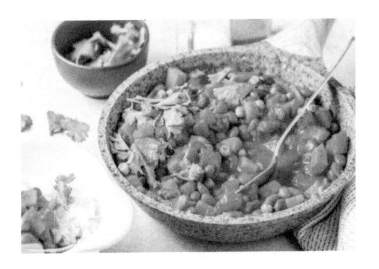

Servings: 8

Ingredients

- 1 Tbsp extra-virgin olive oil

- 1 onion, chopped
- 1 red bell pepper, chopped
- 3 cloves garlic, minced
- 2 pickled jalapeños, finely chopped
- 1 Tbsp tomato paste
- 1 -15.5-oz can pinto beans, drained and rinsed
- 1 -15.5-oz can black beans, drained and rinsed
- 1 -15.5-oz can kidney beans, drained and rinsed
- 1 -28-oz can tomatoes and green chilies
- 3 cups vegetable broth
- 1/4 cup chili powder
- 1/2 tsp cayenne pepper
- 1 Tbsp cumin
- 2 tsp oregano
- kosher salt
- freshly ground black pepper
- cilantro, for serving

Directions

1. In a Dutch oven over medium heat add olive oil. When hot, add onion and red bell pepper and sauté until soft.
2. Add garlic and jalapeno and sauté for 2 minutes.
3. Add tomato paste and stir into vegetables.
4. Add pinto beans, black beans, kidney beans and tomatoes and green chilies and mix together.
5. Add vegetable broth.
6. Add chili powder, cayenne pepper, cumin, oregano and salt and pepper to taste.
7. Bring to a boil and then let simmer for 20 minutes.

8. Serve immediately and top with cilantro.

Optional: top with vegan sour cream and vegan cheese

1. In a large pot over medium heat, heat olive oil then add onion, bell pepper, and carrots. Sauté until soft for about 5 minutes. Add garlic and jalapeño and cook until fragrant, about 1 minute.
2. Add tomato paste and stir to coat vegetables. Add tomatoes, beans, broth, and seasonings. Season with salt and pepper to taste.
3. Bring to a boil then reduce heat and let simmer for about 30 minutes.
4. Serve with cheese, sour cream, and cilantro.

Nutrition

per serving

- Calories 551
- Fat 40 g
- Carbohydrates 51 g
- Protein 7 g

Adapted: delish.com, noracooks.com

VEGETABLE KABOBS

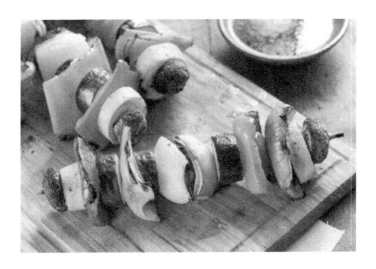

Servings: 6

Ingredients

- 2 cups cremini mushrooms

- 1 cup cherry tomatoes
- 1 red bell pepper, cut into chunks
- 1 green bell pepper, cut into chunks
- 1 red onion, cut into chunks
- 1 green zucchini, sliced into thick rounds
- 1 yellow zucchini, sliced into thick rounds

Marinade

- 1/4 cup olive oil
- 3 cloves garlic, pressed
- Juice of 1 lemon
- 1/2 teaspoon dried oregano
- 1/2 teaspoon dried basil
- kosher salt and freshly ground black pepper, to taste

Directions

1. Preheat the oven to 400°F.
2. In a bowl, whisk together olive oil, garlic, lemon juice, basil, oregano and salt and pepper to taste.
3. Assemble vegetables on a skewer in desired order.
4. Brush vegetables with olive oil mixture.
5. Let vegetables sit for 15 minutes to absorb olive oil mixture.
6. Place skewers in the oven and roast for 10-12 minutes or to desired tenderness. Be careful not to overcook the vegetables.
7. Serve immediately.

Nutrition

- Calories 127.0
- Fat 9.5 g
- Carbohydrates 10 g
- Protein 2.4 g

Adapted: damndelicious.net

VEGAN MINESTRONE SOUP

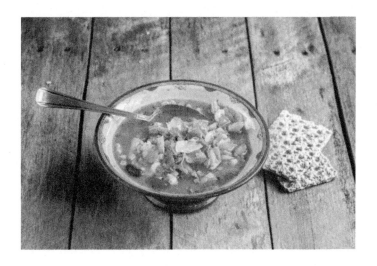

Servings: 4

Ingredients

- 2 Tbsp extra-virgin olive oil

- 1/2 medium yellow onion, diced
- 3 cloves garlic, minced
- 2 large carrots, peeled and sliced into thin rounds
- 1 1/2 cups green beans, trimmed and roughly chopped
- 1/4 tsp each kosher salt & black pepper or more to taste
- 1 small zucchini, sliced into 1/4-inch rounds
- 1 -15-ounce can diced fire-roasted tomatoes
- 6 cups vegetable broth
- 2 tsp dried basil
- 2 tsp dried oregano
- 1 Tbsp nutritional yeast
- 1 pinch red chili pepper flake (optional)
- 1 Tbsp coconut sugar (or other sweetener to taste)
- 1 -15-ounce can chickpeas, rinsed and drained
- 2 cups whole wheat pasta noodles of any shape
- 1 cup spinach or other green, roughly chopped

Directions

1. In a Dutch oven heat oil and add garlic and onions and cook until translucent - about 3 minutes.
2. Add spices and cook for 1 minute.
3. Add carrots, green beans and salt and pepper to taste. Stir and cook until vegetables are soft 3-4 minutes.
4. Add zucchini, tomatoes, vegetables broth,

nutritional yeast, red pepper flakes, coconut sugar and chickpeas. Stir to coat everything.

5. Turn heat to medium-high to achieve a boil. Boil for three minutes and then turn down heat to simmer.

6. Add pasta and cook for 10 more minutes, stir occasionally.

7. Add spinach to soup mixture.

8. Cook for 10 more minutes on a simmer.

9. Turn off heat and let soup cool for a few minutes before serving.

Nutrition

per serving

- Calories: 127
- Fat 2.4 g
- Carbohydrates: 18.1 g
- Protein: 9.2 g

Adapted: minimalistbaker.com

VERY VEGETABLE SOUP

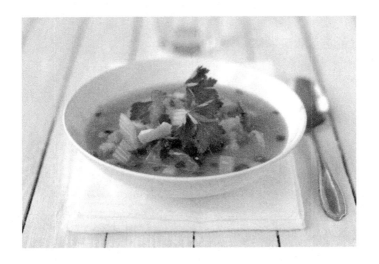

Ingredients

- 2 Tbsp extra virgin olive oil
- 1 large onion, diced
- 3 cloves garlic, minced

- 3 medium carrots, diced
- 3 stalks celery, diced
- 2 medium potatoes, peeled and diced
- 2 tsp Italian seasoning
- 4 cups vegetable broth and 1 cup water
- 2 -15 oz can diced tomatoes
- 1 cup corn
- 1 -15 oz can kidney beans
- 1 bay leaf
- 1/4 cup parsley, chopped
- 1 tbsp freshly squeezed lemon juice, more to taste
- 1 1/2 tsp kosher salt, more to taste
- Freshly ground black pepper

Directions

1. Heat oil in a large Dutch oven over medium heat. Add garlic and onion and sauté until translucent.
2. Add carrots, celery and potatoes and cook for 6 minutes.
3. Add kosher salt and Italian seasoning and cook for 2 minutes.
4. Add broth, pepper, and bay leaf.
5. Add tomatoes, beans, corn, and water.
6. Bring to a boil and then simmer for 20 minutes.
7. Heat oil in a large Dutch oven over medium-low heat. Once hot, add onion, garlic and a teaspoon of kosher salt and cook for about 8 minutes.
8. Remove bay leaf, add parsley and lemon juice.

9. Serve immediately.

Nutrition

- Calories 369
- Fat 9.1 g
- Carbohydrates 56.9 g
- Protein 17.9 g

Adapted: hummusapian.com

WHOLE-WHEAT PASTA SALAD

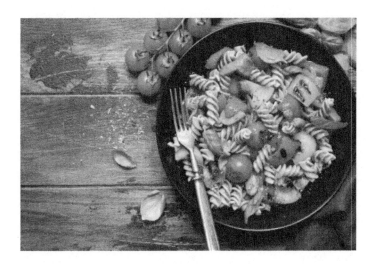

Servings: 8

Ingredients

- 8 ounces dry whole-wheat pasta of any variety
- 4 Tbsp finely chopped fresh basil, divided
- Salt, to taste
- Freshly ground black pepper, to taste
- 1/4 tsp crushed red pepper
- 3 Tbsp extra-virgin olive oil, divided
- 4 cloves garlic, minced and divided
- 1 medium red bell pepper, diced
- 1 cup cherry tomatoes
- 1 cucumber, diced

Directions

1. Cook the pasta according to the package directions.
2. Add salt to water and let water get to a rolling boil.
3. When pasta is done, rinse the pasta, pour it into a bowl, cover, and refrigerate it to cool.
4. In a large mixing bowl, add 2 tablespoons basil, salt, pepper, red pepper, 2 tablespoons oil, and half of the minced garlic and whisk together.
5. Add the cold pasta, bell pepper, cucumber and tomatoes, and toss gently until well coated.
6. Serve immediately.

Nutrition

- Calories 165
- Fat 5.9 g
- Carbohydrate 24.6 g
- Protein 4.7 g

Adapted: godairyfree.org

ZUCCHINI SPAGHETTI

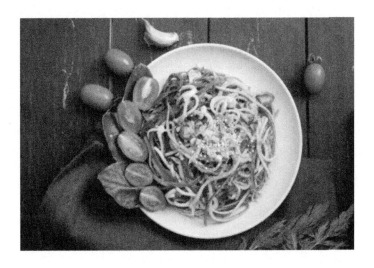

Ingredients

- 2 medium zucchinis, spiralized (see notes below)
- 1/3 cup vegan pesto, plus more if needed
- 1/2 red onion, thinly sliced and halved

- 6 mushrooms, thinly sliced (cremini or white button)
- 10 cherry tomatoes, halved
- 2 cloves garlic, finely minced
- 2 tsp olive oil
- salt, to taste
- freshly ground black pepper (optional)
- red crushed pepper (optional)

Directions

1. Heat the olive oil in a nonstick pan on medium-high heat.
2. Add garlic, onions, and mushrooms. Add about 1/4 teaspoon salt. Cook until vegetables are tender and moisture from mushrooms is cooked away. Set aside mixture on a plate.
3. Clean pan dry.
4. Add 1/4 c. pesto to the heated pan.
5. Add spiralized zucchini and sauté until zucchini is cooked through 1-2 minutes.
6. Add the sautéed onions/mushrooms to the pan.
7. Add tomatoes.
8. Add the rest of the pesto, or more if you want.
9. Sauté for another 1-2 minutes tossing mixture gently.
10. Add red pepper flakes and salt and pepper to taste.

Nutrition

- Calories 266
- Carbohydrates 11.4 g
- Proteins 4.5 g
- Fat 19.6 g

Note: Spiralized Zucchini - you can buy zucchini spiralized, or you can use a special gadget to make it at home.

Adapted: vegetarian gastronomy.com

FINAL WORDS

It is hard to change the way you have been eating all of your life. Unless you had really cool parents who were vegan and they started you on a vegan diet when you were a child, you likely are not that familiar with a whole foods, plant-based diet. To help make the change, you need to keep in mind that a plant-based diet is about adding foods to your diet more than it is about taking something away.

There are many different reasons for abstaining from animal products. Perhaps you care about the environment and what happens to our planet when ranchers raise animals for food. Perhaps you have a personal reason for not eating anything with a face. Whatever the reason that brought you to learning about a plant-based diet, know that from this point on, your health will improve.

Finding plant-based proteins is not as hard as you might think. You might have to adjust to eating tofu and legumes but rest-assured that there are many recipes that feature delicious ways to eat plant-based proteins. In fact, there are curries and stews that can curl your toes with joy and make you happy that you made the change. The trick is to keep an open mind about the changes in your diet. You might miss sugar or having fried foods, but keep in mind that you are doing good for your body.

In this book you learned about choosing whole foods for your diet. Eating foods in their most natural form is a good way to think about eating whole foods. For example, choosing whole wheat foods instead of foods made with enriched flour, or choosing brown rice instead of white rice can help you to avoid the problems that come with eating refined or over-processed foods.

Buying convenience or fast foods brings processed foods into our diet. These foods may be really tasty but they are void and null of the good nutrition that our bodies need. It might be easier to buy fast food when you are in a hurry or to choose convenience foods at the grocery store but are we doing our bodies any favors? In the end, you will develop health problems from depriving your body of the whole foods that it needs.

It is true that changing the way you eat might be tough on your taste buds at first. It's hard to stop eating foods with sugar or lots of salt, but it is possible to get sweetness into your food without reverting to adding sugar. Ripe bananas and dates are a great way to make recipes sweeter. Once you quit sugar and add natural sweetness to your diet, you won't even miss the sugar.

Following a plant-based diet can also help you to lose the

unwanted pounds that you have gained over the years. There are so many diet plans on the market today. Some plans starve you and other plans have you eating nothing but proteins and restricting your carbs. You will find that when you follow a plant-based diet, you lose weight without trying.

The whole foods that you eat on a plant-based diet will fill you up and give you the nutrients that you need. In fact, you will find yourself eating more often instead of starving yourself. It is important to get all your nutrients from your daily diet. Consequently, you will need to eat five times a day to make this happen. Five times a day means that you don't skip any meals and that you add two snacks to your daily meal plans. A plant-based diet will be the only diet that you will need to lose weight and keep that weight off.

As you follow a plant-based diet, you will start to feel a whole lot better than when you were eating junk food and animal products. The health advantages that a plant-based diet may bring to you are lower blood pressure, lower cholesterol, stable blood sugar levels and an energy boost.

Two illnesses that carry serious consequences are cancer and heart disease. Carrying extra weight can put you at risk for these two illnesses. So, as you lose weight on a plant-based diet you decrease your chances of developing cancer or heart disease. The foods that you will be eating on a plant-based diet contribute to your health in ways that you never thought of before.

The Reset Diet and the 14-day Detox Plan are great ways to initiate yourself into plant-based eating and get rid of the toxins that have been collecting in your body. It might have been hard at first to follow the detox plan but I'm sure you felt better once you were done! Feel free to use it anytime you feel that you need to get back to eating a completely plant-based diet.

I'd really like to know what you thought of this book! Is there anything that I can improve on? I worked very hard on this book and would really appreciate it if you could leave me some feedback on how helpful it was for you. You can leave your review on Amazon.

Enjoy your new whole food, plant-based lifestyle!

WORKS CITED

7 Things That Happen When You Stop Eating Meat. (2019, July 02). Retrieved September 02, 2020, from https://www.forksoverknives.com/wellness/7-things-that-happen-when-you-stop-eating-meat/

Beginner's Guide to a Plant-Based Diet. (2020, August 28). Retrieved September 02, 2020, from https://www.forksoverknives.com/how-tos/plant-based-primer-beginners-guide-starting-plant-based-diet/

Blogilates (2017, December 19). 4 Energy Boosting Snack Ideas! Retrieved September 02, 2020, from https://www.blogilates.com/4-energy-boosting-snack-ideas/

Corcoran, C. (2019, June 08). How a Plant-Based Diet Can Boost Energy Levels and Regulate Thyroid Hormones. Retrieved September 02, 2020, from https://www.onegreenplanet.org/natural-health/vegan-plantbased-diet-boosts-energy-regulate-thyroid/

Dolson, L. (2020, March 10). What to Eat on a Whole Foods Diet. Retrieved September 02, 2020, from https://www.verywellfit.com/what-is-a-whole-foods-diet-2241974

Fowler, P., Anonymous. (2015, July 08). Science Says a Plant-Based Diet Is Best for Weight Loss. Retrieved September 02, 2020, from https://www.shape.com/weight-loss/food-weight-loss/why-plant-based-diet-ideal-weight-loss

Frey, M. (2020, March 25). What Is a Plant-Based Diet? Retrieved September 02, 2020, from https://www.verywellfit.com/plant-based-diet-recipes-tips-guidelines-4174728

Holistically Lizzie. (2020, June 29). 7 day rejuvenating vegan meal plan to detox lose weight. Retrieved September 02, 2020, from http://www.holisticallylizzie.com/7-day-rejuvenating-vegan-meal-plan-to-detox-lose-weight/

How much sugar is too much? (n.d.). Retrieved September 02, 2020, from https://www.heart.org/en/healthy-living/healthy-eating/eat-smart/sugar/how-much-sugar-is-too-much

Jager, Matt. (2020, April 14). Reset: 3 Steps To Get Your Plant-Based Diet Back On Track. Retrieved September 02,

2020, from https://www.nomeatathlete.com/plant-based-reset/

Katherine D. McManus, M. (2018, September 27). What is a plant-based diet and why should you try it? Retrieved September 02, 2020, from https://www.health.harvard.edu/blog/what-is-a-plant-based-diet-and-why-should-you-try-it-2018092614760

Kesseli, P. (2020, January 20). Why You Should Think Twice About a Plant-Based Diet. Retrieved September 02, 2020, from https://mealpreponfleek.com/think-twice-plant-based-diet/

Kubala, J. (n.d.). Whole-Foods, Plant-Based Diet: A Detailed Beginner's Guide. Retrieved September 02, 2020, from https://www.healthline.com/nutrition/plant-based-diet-guide

Lawler, M., Migala, J., Rapaport, L., Delzo, J. (n.d.). 9 Scientific Benefits of Following a Plant-Based Diet: Everyday Health. Retrieved September 02, 2020, from https://www.everydayhealth.com/diet-nutrition/scientific-benefits-following-plant-based-diet/

Lawler, M., Migala, J., Rapaport, L., & Delzo, J. (n.d.). Beginner's Guide to a Plant-Based Diet: Food List, Meal Plan, Benefits, and More: Everyday Health. Retrieved September 02, 2020, from https://www.everydayhealth.com/diet-nutrition/plant-based-diet-food-list-meal-plan-benefits-more/

Lawler, M., Migala, J., Rapaport, L., Delzo, J. (n.d.). Plant-Based Diet: Food List and 14-Day Sample Menu: Everyday Health. Retrieved September 02, 2020, from https://www.everydayhealth.com/diet-nutrition/plant-based-diet-food-list-sample-menu/

Lingel, Grant (2019, December 17). Veganism: 20 Powerful Reasons You Should Go Vegan. Retrieved September 02, 2020, from https://sentientmedia.org/veganism/Losing Weight on a Plant-Based, Vegan Diet: Tips for Success. (2019, December 20). Retrieved September 02, 2020, from https://www.forksoverknives.com/how-tos/vegan-plant-based-diet-weight-loss-diet-tips/

MD Anderson Cancer Center, Alexander, H. (2019, December 10). 5 benefits of a plant-based diet. Retrieved September 02, 2020, from https://www.mdanderson.org/publications/focused-on-health/5-benefits-of-a-plant-based-diet.h20-1592991.html

Minimalistbaker (2020, May 25). Healthy Smoothie Recipes: Minimalist Baker Recipes. Retrieved September 02, 2020, from https://minimalistbaker.com/12-simple-healthy-smoothie-ideas/

MS, M. (2020, June 23). The Body Reset Diet: Does It Work for Weight Loss? Retrieved September 02, 2020, from https://www.healthline.com/nutrition/body-reset-diet

Mucerino, C. (2020, July 24). Join a Plant Based Party This Weekend By Eating One Vegan Meal. Retrieved September 02, 2020, from https://thebeet.com/give-back-to-support-feed-and-reverb-by-eating-one-vegan-meal-this-weekend/

Nagesh, A. (2018, November 23). Brace yourselves - these nine things aren't actually vegan - BBC Three. Retrieved September 02, 2020, from https://www.bbc.co.uk/bbcthree/article/578edf2d-9c22-453e-ab33-48f7a0568c0b

Petre, A. (2016, September 23). 6 Science-Based Health Benefits of Eating Vegan. Retrieved September 02, 2020, from https://www.healthline.com/nutrition/vegan-diet-benefits

Petre, A. (n.d.). The 17 Best Protein Sources For Vegans and Vegetarians. Retrieved September 02, 2020, from https://www.healthline.com/nutrition/protein-for-vegans-vegetarians

Plant-based diets can remedy chronic diseases. (2012, October 17). Retrieved September 02, 2020, from https://www.sciencedaily.com/releases/2012/10/121017131546.htm

Seaver, V. (n.d.). 7-Day Vegetarian Meal Plan: 1,200 Calories. Retrieved September 02, 2020, from http://www.eatingwell.com/article/288729/7-day-vegetarian-meal-plan-1200-calories/

Spalding, L. (2013, February 15). Plant-Based Eating: The Benefits of Cleaning Up Your Diet. Retrieved September 02, 2020, from https://www.yogajournal.com/lifestyle/crunch-time

Vegetarian diet: How to get the best nutrition. (2020, August 20). Retrieved September 02, 2020, from https://www.mayoclinic.org/healthy-lifestyle/nutrition-and-healthy-eating/in-depth/vegetarian-diet/art-20046446

Why Oil-Free? (n.d.). Retrieved September 02, 2020, from https://nakedfoodmagazine.com/why-oil-free/

Why Salt-free? (n.d.). Retrieved September 02, 2020, from https://nakedfoodmagazine.com/why-salt-free/